# Maternal and Child Health Matters Around the World

*Edited by Masoud Mohammadnezhad and Nafisa Huq*

Published in London, United Kingdom

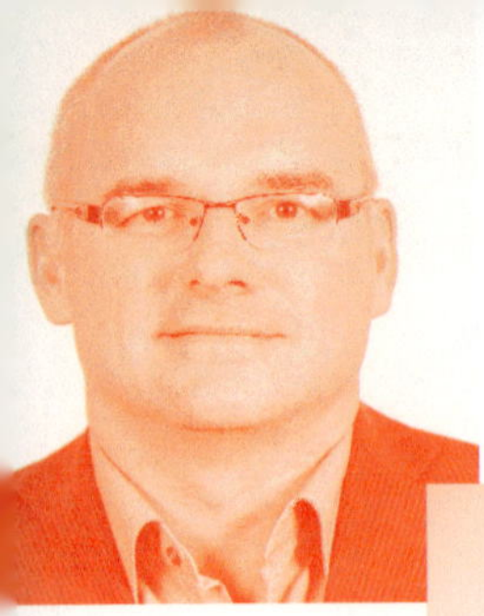
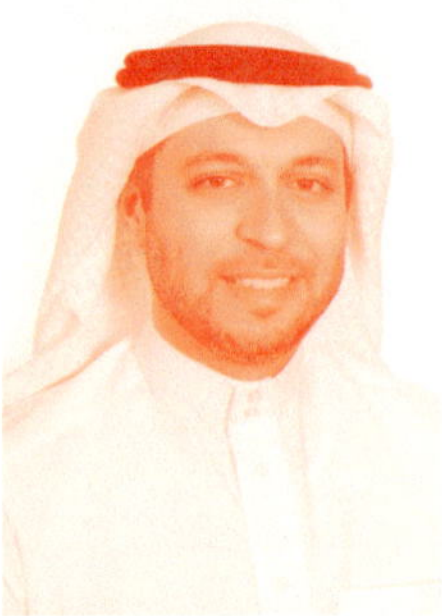
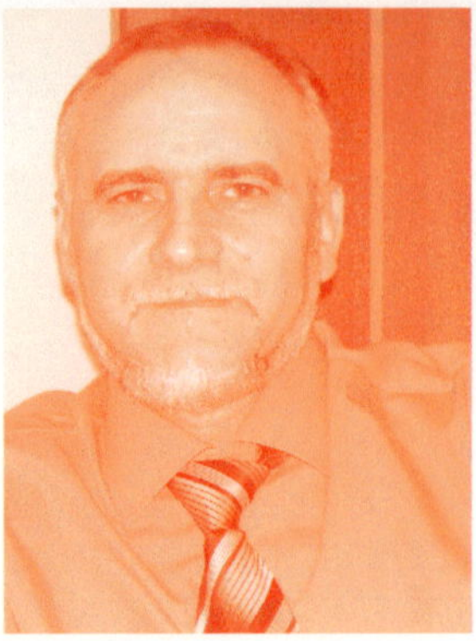
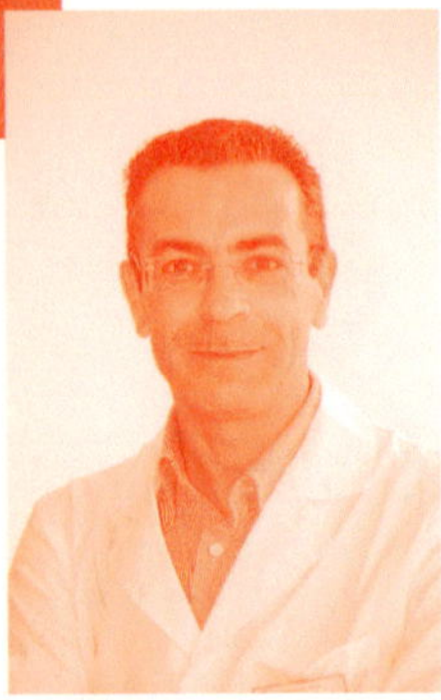
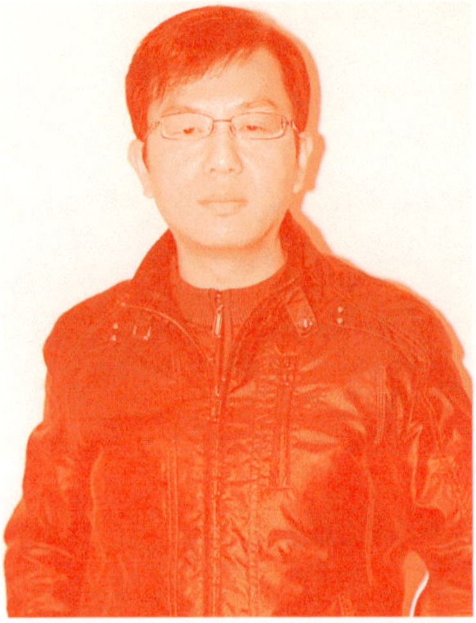
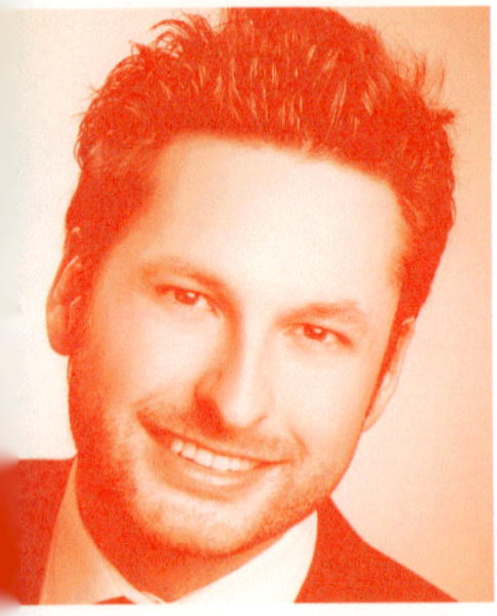
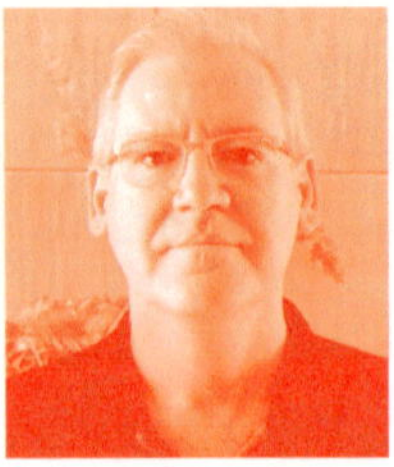

IntechOpen

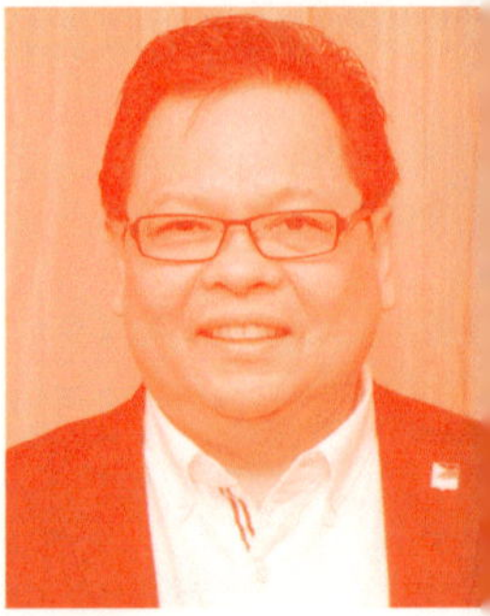
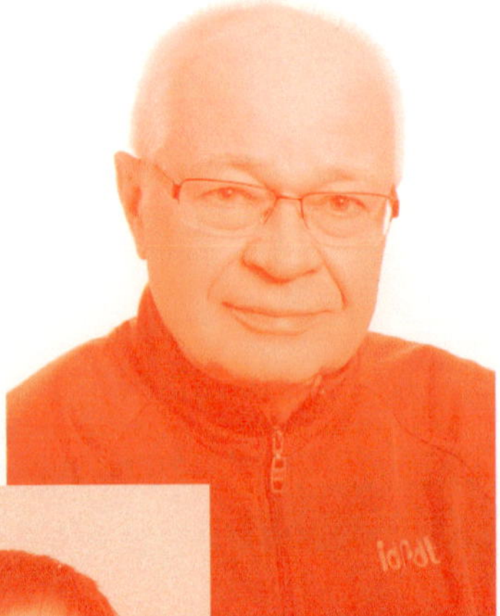
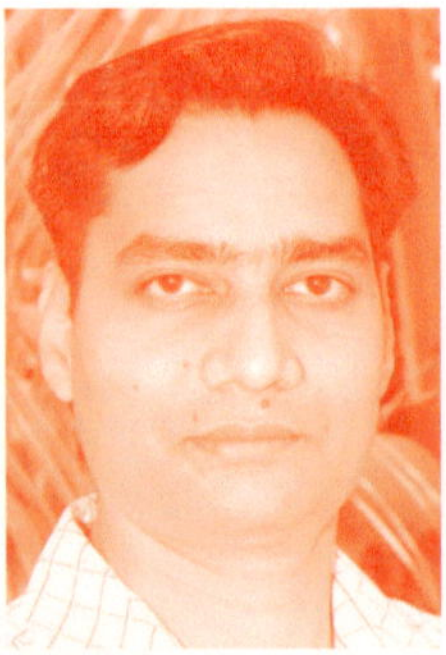
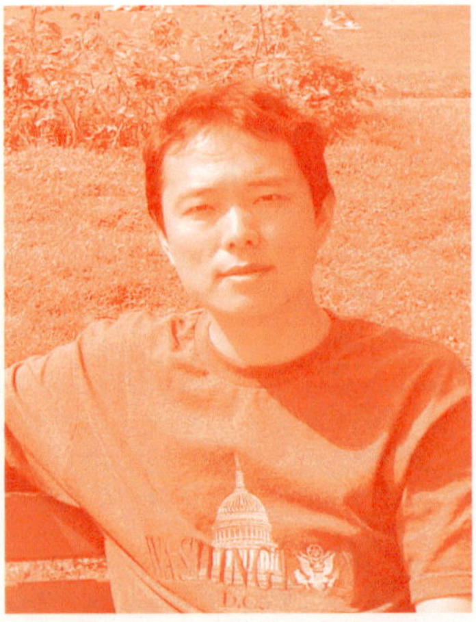
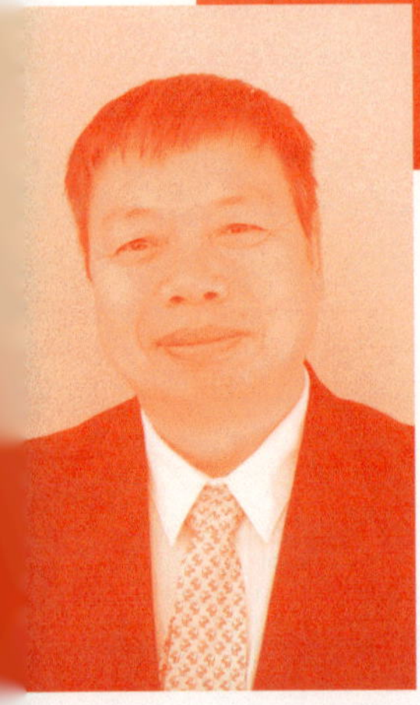
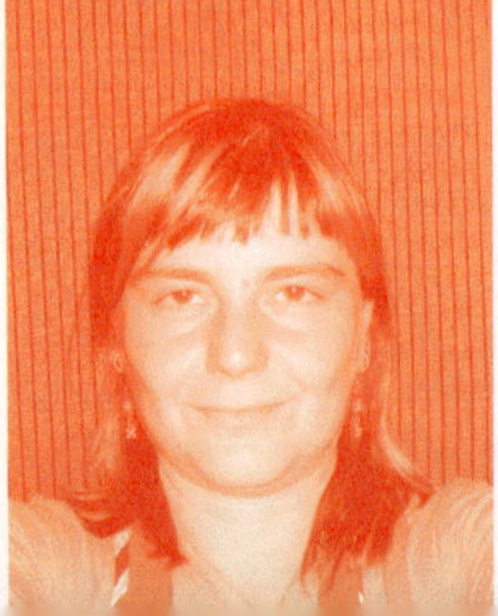

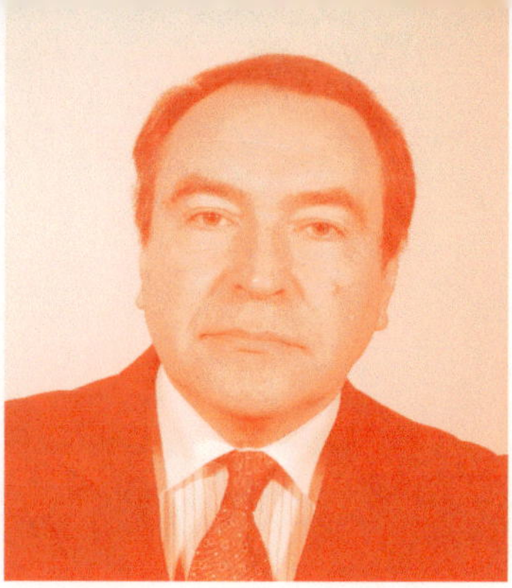
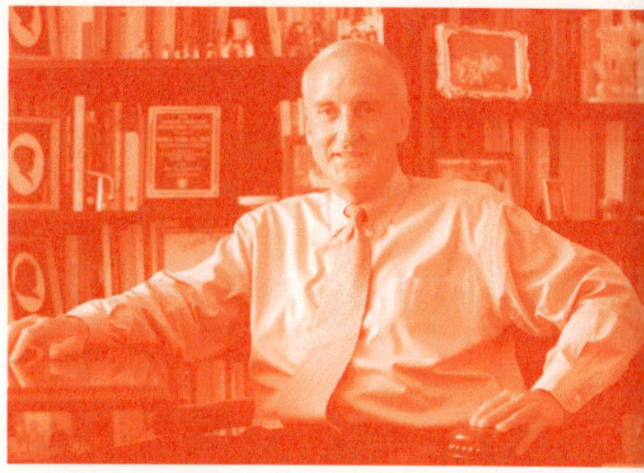
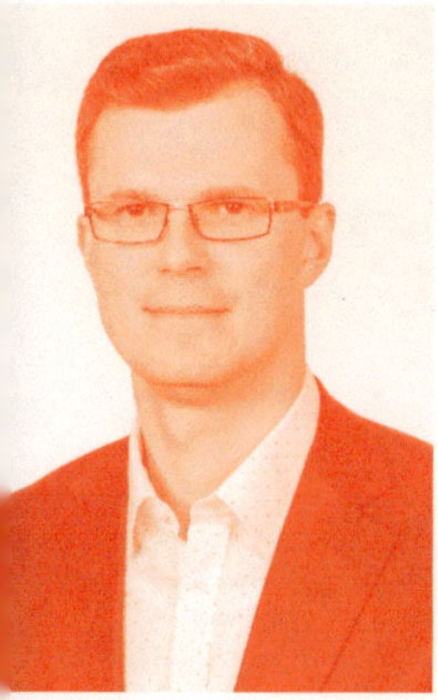
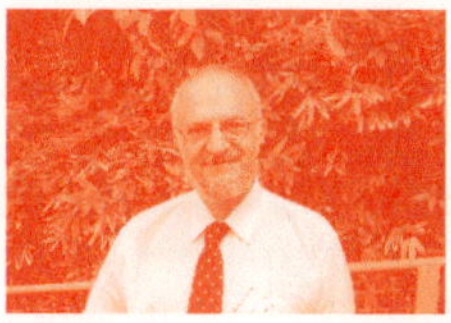
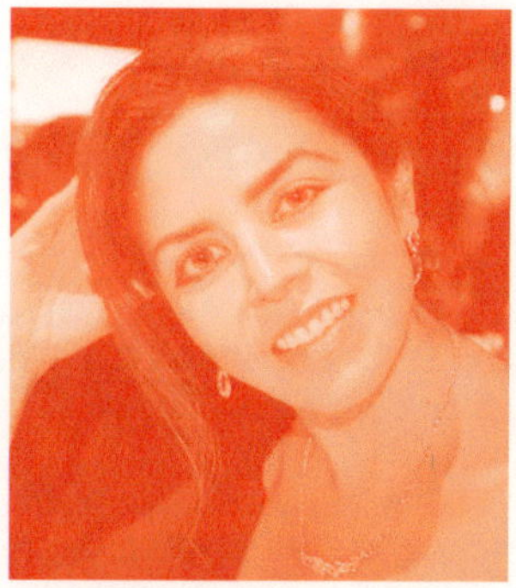

*Supporting open minds since 2005*

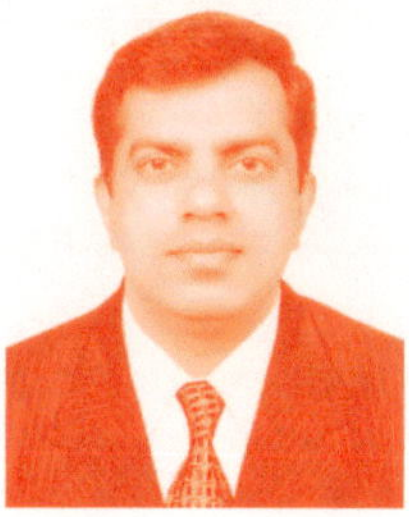
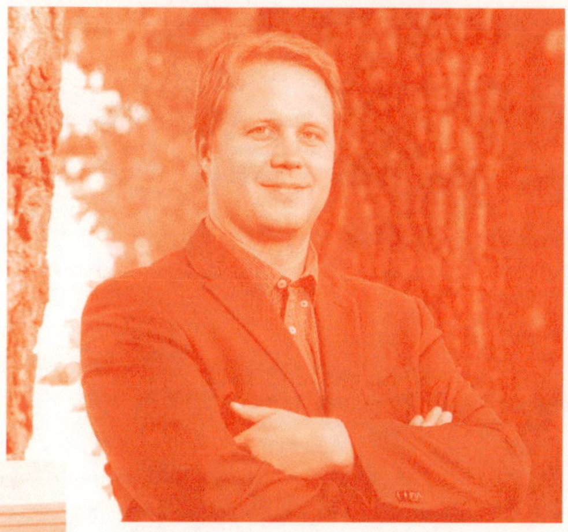
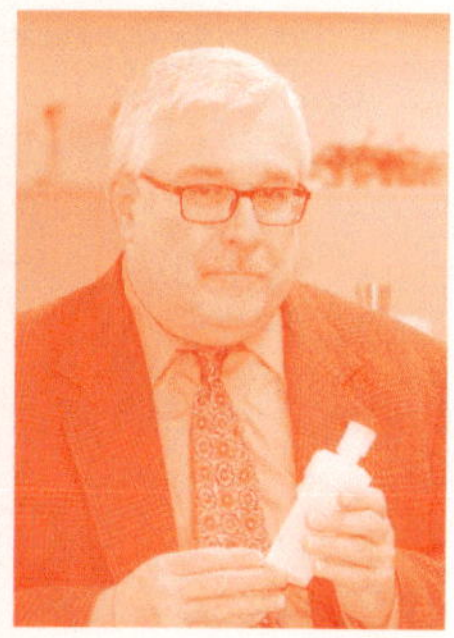
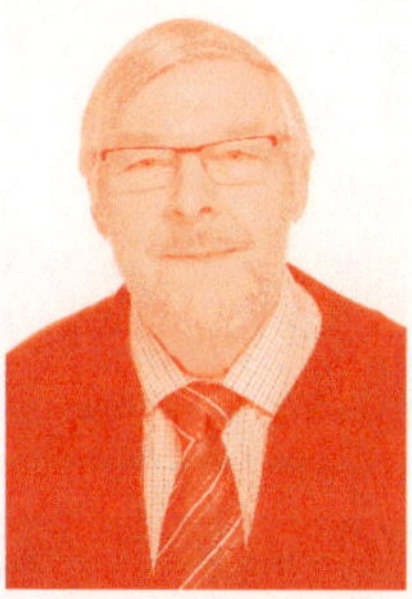
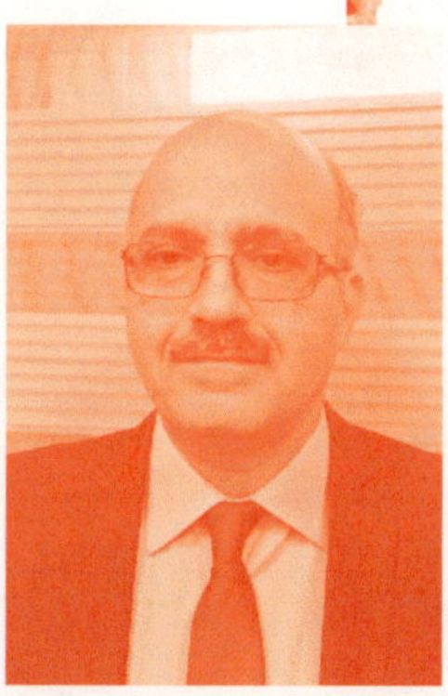
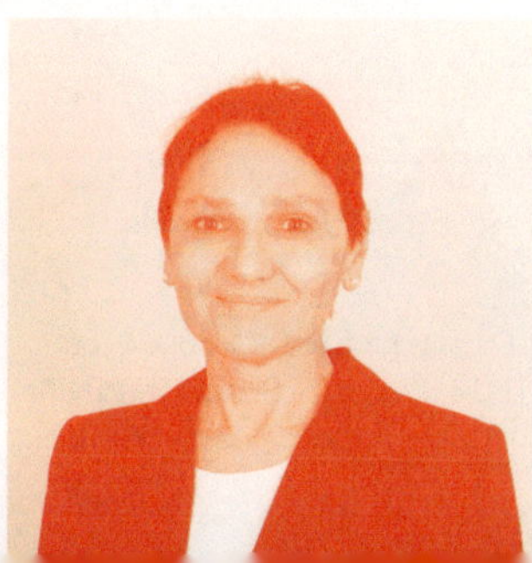
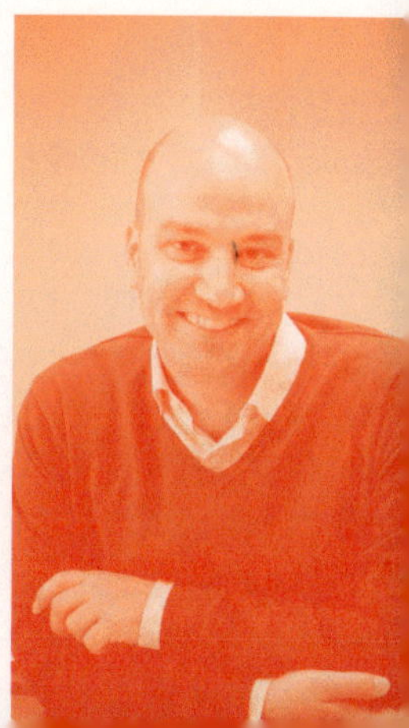

Maternal and Child Health Matters Around the World
http://dx.doi.org/10.5772/intechopen.78255
Edited by Masoud Mohammadnezhad and Nafisa Huq

Contributors
Navaneetham Janardhana, Elena Nikolaeva, Vera Merenkova, Aline Mizutani Gomes, Renato Alves, Luis Peña-Quintana, Yessica Rodriguez-Santana, Rayhan SK, Somdutta Barua, Jean-Baptiste Kakoma, Xavier Kinenkinda, Fanny Malonga, Joseph Nsambi, Micrette Ngalula, Jeanne Ngoy, Jean Kalibushi, Bonifacio Caballero-Noguez, Ernesto Calderon Cisneros, Roberto Aguli Ruíz Rosas, Basavaraj Manjula



First published in London, United Kingdom, 2020 by IntechOpen
IntechOpen is the global imprint of INTECHOPEN LIMITED, registered in England and Wales, registration number: 11086078, 7th floor, 10 Lower Thames Street, London, EC3R 6AF, United Kingdom
Printed in Croatia

British Library Cataloguing-in-Publication Data
A catalogue record for this book is available from the British Library

Additional hard and PDF copies can be obtained from orders@intechopen.com

Maternal and Child Health Matters Around the World
Edited by Masoud Mohammadnezhad and Nafisa Huq
p. cm.
Print ISBN 978-1-83968-379-4
Online ISBN 978-1-83968-380-0
eBook (PDF) ISBN 978-1-83968-381-7

For EU product safety concerns:
IN TECH d.o.o., Prolaz Marije Krucifikse Kozulić 3, 51000 Rijeka, Croatia, info@intechopen.com or visit our website at intechopen.com.

# Meet the editors

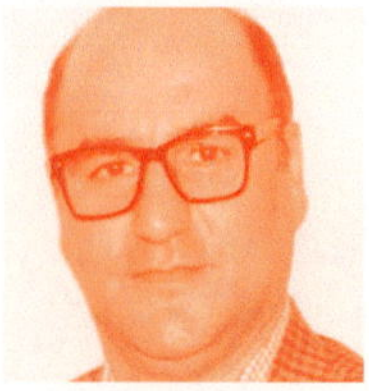

Dr. Masoud Mohammadnezhad graduated with a MSc in Health Promotion from Tarbiat Modares University in Iran in 2002 and was awarded his Ph.D. in Public Health from Flinders University, Australia, in 2014. Dr Mohammadnezhad has more than 15 years of experience in teaching undergraduate, postgraduate, and MBBS courses in various university settings. He is currently teaching a variety of public health courses, along with developing the course outlines, at Fiji National University (FNU), where he is an Associate Professor of Public Health (Health Promotion) in the School of Public Health and Primary Care, along with being the program coordinator for the health promotion discipline. He has published more than 50 articles, seven of which have been published in 2017. He has published more than 70 articles and have also presented at more than 60 national and international conferences. He is an editorial board member of several leading international journals, such as Global Health Journal, and a reviewer for a number of high quality journals, such as the British Medical Journal, BMC Public Health, PLOS ONE, Rural and Remote Health, Health Promotion Journal of Australia, and Journal of Clinical Nursing.

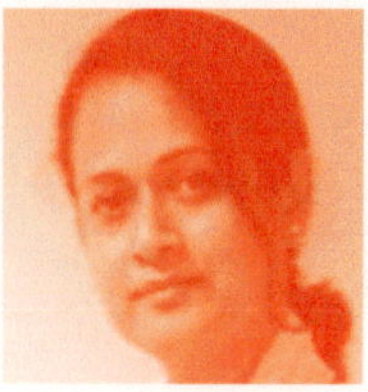

Dr. Nafisa Huq is an academician and health care professional working in the School of Public Health, Independent University, Bangladesh. Alongside teaching graduate and undergraduate courses, she is responsible for assisting in research projects at the university and undertaking some administrative duties. Her research interest is in community mental health with a special focus on women and children. Mental health is a significant part of health that influences other aspects of maternal and child health especially with regard to nutrition, self-care, child care, and education. She has recently completed field work on a fellowship from the South Asian Hub for Advocacy Research and Education (SHARE) in mental health where she looked into health care seeking behavior of rural women with and without depression. She also works with Mental Health Awareness Training Education and Research (MATERS) Trust where one of the goals is to address persistent disparities in maternal, infant, and child health with a "life course" perspective to health promotion and disease prevention.

# Contents

# Preface

This edited volume is a collection of reviewed and relevant research chapters, concerning the latest developments within the maternal and child health matters around the world field of study. The book includes scholarly contributions by various authors and has been edited by a group of medical experts.

Each contribution comes as a separate chapter complete in itself but directly related to the book's topics and objectives.

There are 7 chapters in this book and they are as follows:

CHAPTER 1: The Interrelation of the Mother's Health Status with the State of Health of First- and Second-Year-Old Children

CHAPTER 2: Public Policies for Promotion of Maternal-Infant Health in Brazil: Some Experiences with Adolescent Mothers in São Paulo

CHAPTER 3: Cytokines and Maternal Omega-3 LCPUFAs Supplementation

CHAPTER 4: Correlates of Caesarean Section Delivery in West Bengal, India: An Analysis Based on DLHS-3

CHAPTER 5: Safe Childbirth and Motherhood in African Great Lakes Region: External Pelvimetry in Nulliparae and Scheduled Caesarean Section

CHAPTER 6: Quality Care for Mothers and Newborns at Birth in Mexico

CHAPTER 7: Adolescents Romantic Relationship: Dynamics of Parent-Child Relationship from India

The target audience comprises scholars and specialists in the field.

**IntechOpen**

Chapter 1

# The Interrelation of the Mother's Health Status with the State of Health of First- and Second-Year-Old Children

*Elena Nikolaeva and Vera Merenkova*

## Abstract

We evaluated the state of health of the mother and child at birth, and the probability of the diagnosis of cancelation in the child at the end of the second year of life. The sample consisted of 100 mother-child dyads. The complex assessment of the children's health status was based on the individual medical records. Mothers filled the questionnaire evaluating the mother's relation to her child during the first 2 years of life, and the questionnaire aimed at assessing the emotional intelligence level. Almost all the children at birth have one or the other diagnosis. There is a positive connection between the number of the diagnoses in the first- and second-year-old children during their stay in the maternity ward and perinatal pathology factors of the mother. But by the end of the second year of life in 60% of the children, these diagnoses were canceled. The healthier the mother, the more positive the prognosis with regard to the child's health within the first 2 years of living is. Positive prognosis with regard to the first-year-old children's health depends upon the acceptance of the child by the mother: the higher the value on the scale of acceptance-nonacceptance is, the better the child's health is.

**Keywords:** dyad mother-child, health, emotional intelligence, attachment, perinatal pathology, encephalopathy, Russia

## 1. Introduction

Man's health is an essential condition of his/her wellbeing, self-fulfillment and an active creation [1, 2]. However, throughout the world, there is a great number of people suffering from different diseases. A part of them is connected with the process of gestating and bearing a child, many of them are a result of poverty, and some others are a consequence of aging [3]. Nowadays, many scientists define the reason for hereditary disease growth as a result of that mankind has gone out of control of natural selection. For instance, at the end of the nineteenth century in Russia, 85% of infants who were born in summer died [4]. The reason for most children's death was intestinal infections and mothers' employment in agricultural works that decreased their care for the child. At present, infant mortality has fallen, but a lot of diseases have emerged. They may be an effect during pregnancy, some chronic diseases have exacerbates in the mother, or she has had infectious diseases, experienced the acute stress, etc. The mother for the child is a natural environment in the course of development, and her health, of course, determines his/her health. Maternal organism provides everything the child needs in and develops in [5].

### 1.1 The mother's diseases during the pregnancy and the child's health

The extragenital and chronic genital pathology exerts a significant influence upon pregnancy outcome for the fetus [6]. Among the factors of adverse effect on the fetus, researchers point out chronic hypoxia due to the disturbance of utero-placental blood circulation, the sympathetic-adrenal system insufficiency, fetal growth retardation, immaturity, the disturbance of function of cardiovascular and respiratory systems. Consequently, there appears a risk of the premature termination of pregnancy and birth of a premature baby [7]. Fetoplacental insufficiency is a complex of disturbances of placenta functions (transport, trophic, endocrine and metabolic) caused by morphofunctional changes in it and utero-placental blood circulation disturbance [8]. Placental insufficiency is a cause of the development disturbance and intrauterine hypoxia of the fetus and pathological statuses and diseases of a newborn baby.

At present, fetal hypoxia occupies a leading place in the structure of the reasons for perinatal mortality (from 40 to 70%) as well as central nervous system impairments in the fetus or a newborn (from 30 to 80%), which in turn lead to different disturbances of the somatic and neuromental development of children. At that, the degree of the severity of these pathological deviations depends upon the duration and severity of intrauterine hypoxia [9]. The chronic fetal hypoxia, fetal infection and birth trauma are main reasons for the perinatal lesion of central nervous system and the strongest stress factor [10, 11]. Fetoplacental insufficiency may arise throughout pregnancy but complications for the fetus manifest mainly during the third trimester. At delivery, fetal asphyxia progresses often in mothers with chronic fetoplacental insufficiency. The reason for that is an acute and chronic hypoxia of the fetus [12]. Newborn children have the central nervous system disturbances, changes in reflex excitability, cyanosis, bradycardia and so on [13]. The newborn children, whose mothers suffer from fetoplacental insufficiency, are born in the state of severe asphyxia in 10% of cases, and 81% experience a pathological course of an early neonatal period [14, 15].

In Russia, maternal toxemia during the first half of pregnancy occurs in 50% of women, late toxicosis in 2–30% of pregnant and parturient women [16]. Late gestosis represent a symptom complex of multiorgan and multisystem insufficiency, which manifest clinically more often from the 20th week of pregnancy and end immediately at birth or later after delivery [15]. The disturbances of mental, emotional and physical development are found in 20% of newborns from mothers with late gestosis; child morbidity rises considerably [17].

A number of investigations have shown that children born after pregnancy with gestosis have perinatal brain lesion, neurological complications, dysontogenesis, physical and neuromental development retardation, minimal brain dysfunction and immature indices of electroencephalogram [18]. Premature discharge of amniotic fluid is considered as an amniotic fluid release due to the rupture of membranes before the beginning of childbirth regardless of duration of gestation [19]. About 35% of premature labor is accompanied by premature discharge of amniotic fluid [20].

Among risk factors of premature discharge of amniotic fluid, there are aborts in an anamnesis (48%), inflammatory processes of genitals (33%), extragenital infectious diseases (12%), anomalies of the bone pelvis (8.5%) and hydramnion (3.4%). In case of premature discharge of amniotic fluid, complications during the childbirth and postpartum period increase considerably: birth abnormalities

(16%), bleeding during the postpartum and early postpartum periods (12.5%) and so on [21, 22].

The growth of the incidence of dystocia is explained by the increase of a number of reasons leading to the development of that pathology. Central nervous system dysfunction underlies dystocia, namely: disturbance of equilibrium of the sympathetic and parasympathetic divisions, somatic and genital diseases, endocrine disorders, flat fetal bladder and discrepancy between the fetus size and the mother's pelvis. Quite often, the reason for that anomaly is an undue and untimely prescription of stimulating-delivery remedies [23].

Among the peculiarities of neonatal period in children from mothers with weakness of labor activity, there is a decrease of a favorable outcome of early adaption by newborns alongside with the prevalence of the perinatal lesion of central nervous system [24]. In many works, one points out a considerable influence of risk factors during the pre- and perinatal periods on the development of the cerebrum on the whole and higher cortical functions, which enhance the heterochrony of functional systems maturation [25]. The influence of the health of pregnant women on the somatic and mental health of infants is out of doubt. However, it is noteworthy that the totality of data evidence that in the long run, the mother's diseases lead to an inadequate nutrition of a baby in the course of gestation and oxygen anoxemia. During the antenatal and, particularly, postnatal periods, again, the influence of the mental health of the mother on the mental health of children is less obvious and mediated, as it involves both genetic and environmental factors.

### 1.2 The mother-child dyad after birth

After birth, the child is connected with the mother physiologically and psychologically. During the first two living years, the mother's influence on his or her development almost overlaps all the other factors [26]. Even if the child gets any diagnosis at birth, in many cases there may come recovery under the adequate care of him or her [27]. The child's brain is extremely flexible during the first year of life that is why even traumas can be jugulated under quality care of him or her [28]. According to the modern concepts, the emotional connection between the child beginning from the first years of life and the mother is a major factor of his/her healthy development [29]. One should accept that it is the mother who is a main source of signs forming the emotional-informative environment of the child at early stages of his life [30].

According to Bowlby [31], a close relationship forms between the child and an adult caring during the first 2 years. They are built on the basis of the mutual direction to each other: the child seeks the contact, and the mother responds to it. That kind of behavior is determined biologically and is reasonable evolutionally, since in early days after birth, the child has to find the one who will defend and guard him [32]. According to the theory of attachment, the quality of the formed attachment depends directly on the child's parent who may take care of him in a different way. Ainsworth with co-authors [33] observed the communication of 26 mothers and their children aged one and a half years old during 1 year. As an indicator of attachment, they evaluated the child's behavior at the moment of the mother's arrival and departure.

Based on the observations, three types of children's reactions are described, which correspond to three types of attachment of the child to the mother. Ainsworth calls them anxious-avoidant (A), secure (B) and anxious-resistant or ambivalent (C) types.

The important thing is that children with secure attachment grow into adults who will care for their health and take the responsibility for that. On the contrary, children brought up under the circumstances of insecure attachment often grow into people depending on pernicious habits [34]. The emotional behavior of the mother is predetermined considerably by her emotional intelligence [35–38]. The ability to realize and ponder over one's own and others' emotions, of course, implies numerous consequences, first of all, in a person's behavior. Due to that, the interrelation between emotional intelligence and attachment degree is of absolute interest [29, 33, 39, 40]. This is especially significant, since attachment involves the phenomena, which in the real life a person verbalizes seldom. It is difficult to imagine the mother who says by herself: "I accept my child", or "I support and I do not ignore my child". Attachment to the child is an intimate feeling being close to the instinct [31], and a person does not speak to himself or herself about its details.

We assume that one of the most important parameters influencing the child's health is a level of the emotional maturity of the mother. It manifests in the high emotional intelligence and emotional attachment to the child. We set the task to evaluate the state of health of the mother and child at birth, and the probability of the diagnosis cancelation in the child at the end of the second year of life. It depends upon two characteristics of the mother: emotional intelligence and the degree of attachment to the child.

In Russia, quality examination of the child is fulfilled after birth in the maternity hospital, and a major part of children gets one or the other diagnosis. Another attending doctor may cancel the diagnosis of the child, if the child's status has been normalized. At that, by the end of the first and, quite often, second year of life, medical specialists cancel children's diagnoses made earlier [27]. To a considerable extent, the child's status change is determined by efficient actions of caring persons, mainly, the mother [41]. It is the mother who in the majority of families takes the child to a doctor and carries out all the necessary directions for the rehabilitation. In that situation, her involvement in the process of the child's health recovery impacts substantially on the positive prediction of his/her recovery provided that the disease is not genetic but determined by the peculiarities of intrauterine development and birth.

## 2. Materials and methods

### 2.1 Sample

The sample consisted of 100 mother-child dyads. There were 48 girls, 52 boys and 100 mothers. Among children, there were 50 children aged under 1-year-old (27 boys and 23 girls) and 50 children at the age of 1–2 years old (25 boys and 25 girls).

The experimental sample was selected by means of randomization, that is, by the random selection strategy or subjects distribution when all the subjects had an equal chance to enter the group. It provided internal validity and controlled the blending effect. The present study was carried out in an urban polyclinic for children in a little town of the European part of Russia.

### 2.2 Measures

The complex assessment of the children's health status was based on the individual medical records. The mothers filled the questionnaire evaluating the mother's relation to her child during the first 2 years of life [42] and the questionnaire aimed at assessing the emotional intelligence level [43]. The questionnaire evaluating the mother's relation to her child includes four scales: sensitivity-insensitivity; attachment-rejection; support-ignoring and efficiency-intervention. The questionnaire assessing emotional intelligence level includes three scales: interpersonal emotional intelligence (EI), intrapersonal EI, emotions understanding, emotion management, some subscales and aggregate indicator of EI. It was showed earlier that both questionnaires were valid and reliable [42, 43].

The complex assessment of the children's state of health was based on six main indicators (criteria) of health [16]. These indicators are used by all doctors in the state clinics in Russia for child health assessment. We used the results of the doctor's assessments from the individual records of the children. The first criterion: peculiarities of ontogeny (individual development) described according to the genealogical, biological and social anamnesis. The second criterion: a degree of physical development and its harmoniousness. The physical development of the child was assessed by means of the comparison of individual indicators (body length and weight, chest circumference, etc.) and age standards. At that, body length was the most informative and leading feature in the evaluation of physical development. It was important not only to solve the question of correspondence of the physical development indicators of the child to his/her age but also to assess the harmoniousness of his/her development.

The third criterion: a level of nervous and mental development of the child depends upon both central nervous system state of the child, musculoskeletal system and the environment effect.

The fourth criterion: a level of organism resistance assessed by the quantity of acute diseases during the year preceding the examination. According to this criterion, the children were divided into two groups: with good resistance of organism (having had no diseases during a year, or having had diseases from one to three times); with a lower resistance of organism (having had diseases more than four times a year). The fifth criterion: a level of the functional state of organism based on the aggregate of results of laboratory and instrumental examinations of the child (pulse rate, breath, hemoglobin content in the blood and so on), analysis of his or her behavior and adaptive capabilities. The mother accumulated knowledge about the child's behavior during everyday contact with him or her. The following parameters were assessed during the observation of the child: emotional state, mood, sleep, wake, appetite and the nature of relationships with children and adults, at an older age—the ability to concentrate, attention and fatigability. It was important to take into account individual peculiarities of behavior.

The sixth criterion: the presence or absence of chronic diseases or congenital malformation.

Based on the complex assessment of the above-mentioned criteria, five groups of health were distinguished:

Group I: healthy children having no abnormalities according to all the six criteria.

Group II-A: children having abnormalities according to the first criterion only (ontogeny peculiarities).

Group II-B: children having some functional disorders (including behavior), physical and/or nervous and mental developmental disturbances (or without any of them) and frequent illnesses.

Group III: children having chronic diseases at the stage of compensation, that is, without any disorders of health.

Group IV: children having chronic diseases exacerbating 2–4 times per year, at the stage of subcompensation.

Group V: children having chronic diseases at the stage of decompensation.

### 2.3 Research techniques

We received permits from the children's parents to use the information from their individual medical records. Mothers with children went to the doctor (in Russia mothers of the first-year-old children show their children to the doctors each months) and filled in the questionnaires when the doctor analyzed the health of the child. Then they showed the doctor's records for the researchers. They received the psychological consultations if they participate in the investigation.

For the statistical analysis, the program SPSS-22 was used.

## 3. Results and discussion

The analysis of the data about the pregnancy of the mothers having first- and second-year-old children showed the following results. About 62% of the mothers of first-year-old children and 66% of the mothers of second-year-old children had a first pregnancy. About 26% of the women had a second one. A total of 6% of the mothers of children aged under one-year-old and 2% of the mothers of children at the age of 1–2 years old had a third pregnancy; 4 and 2% correspondingly—a fourth and fifth one, and as little as 1% of the mothers of second-year-old children had a sixth pregnancy.

Interpreting the data about planned and unintended pregnancy, it was noteworthy that the child was "planned and desired" for 72% of the mothers of first-year-old children and 62% of the mothers of second-year-old children. The baby was "unexpected but desired" for 28 and 38% of the women correspondingly. At that, the majority of the mothers (72%), having children aged less than 2 years old, experienced joy, having learned about their pregnancy. Thus, the total sample consisted of 200 subjects under test; there were 50 dyads of "the mother-the first-year-old child" (mean age of the mothers is 24.5 ± 5.6 years old) and 50 dyads of "the mother-the second-year-old child" (mean age of the mothers is 25.5 ± 4.9 years old).

### 3.1 Description of health peculiarities in the children during the first 2 years of life

Based on **Table 1**, in the maternity hospital, the first-year-old children at the moment of examination get approximately the same number of diagnoses: two ones per child on the average. During the first year of living, the number of diagnoses diminishes; and there is one diagnosis per two second-year-old children. That fall of incidence is statistically significant. There are no significant differences in these parameters for the boys and girls.

In spite of the incidence fall, valid differences in the number of the children in the different groups of health at the first and second years of life are not found. This is accounted for that many second-year-old children are identified as group 2A. It includes the children who have no diseases and are almost healthy except these or other peculiarities of the anamnesis at the present moment. As described further, almost all of them have abnormalities owing exactly to the biological anamnesis of the mother.

The obtained results required a more in-depth consideration of morbidity (**Table 2**). The data (in %), obtained and presented in **Table 2**, show that the most widespread diseases are intrauterine hypoxia and physiological jaundice diagnosed in the children during their stay in the maternity ward. Almost all the children have one or the other disease at birth (90% of the first-year-old children, 96% of the second-year-old children). By the end of the first year of life, the diagnoses are canceled in 40% of the children, and in 60% of the children during the second year of life.

| Parameters | The number of diagnosis | | | | | |
|---|---|---|---|---|---|---|
| | The first-year-old children | | | The second-year-old children | | |
| | All children | Girls | Boys | All children | Girls | Boys |
| The number of diagnoses made in the maternity hospital | 2.0 ± 1.1 | 2.0 ± 1.1 | 2.2 ± 1.0 | 2.4 ± 1.5 | 2.6 ± 1.7 | 2.2 ± 1.3 |
| The number of diagnosis made by a local doctor | 1.2 ± 1.1 | 1.2 ± 1.1 | 1.2 ± 1.2 | 0.6 ± 0.9** | 0.8 ± 0.9 | 0.7 ± 1.0 |

**Differences between of the first and second old children* $p = 0.95$.
** $p = 0.99$ *(there and late* T*-criterion).*

**Table 1.**
*The number of diagnosis of the children made in the maternity hospital and by local doctors.*

The data, obtained and presented in **Table 2**, show that the most widespread diseases are intrauterine hypoxia and physiological jaundice diagnosed in the children during their stay in the maternity ward. Almost all the children have one or the other disease at birth (90% of the first-year-old children, 96% of the second-year-old children). By the end of the first year of life, the diagnoses are canceled in 40% of the children, and in 60% of the children during the second year of life. These disorders are the typical one during pregnancy in many countries [3, 15, 21, 24, 44, 45]. This is a typical distribution of neonatal morbidity in Russia [12, 41].

In **Table 3**, there are data about the number of canceled and non-canceled diagnoses for each of the diseases made by a local doctor earlier during the first 2 years. It is evident that during the second year of life already, a major part of the children come to the healthy group (retaining health group II-A because of the burdened anamnesis). There are no differences in this parameter between the boys and girls.

Thus, after the analysis of the medical histories of the children, one can say that the percentage of the healthy children at birth is very small. But the situation changes substantially during the first 2 years of living: a major part of the children's diagnoses are canceled by a local doctor. That is why it is highly important to explore the reasons, which enhance the probability of recovery during the most flexible period of the child's life.

### 3.2 The interrelation of the biological anamnesis of the mother with the health of the first- and second-year-old children

By the end of the first 2 years of life, a major part of the children passes to the group of healthy children. There appears a question of particular peculiarities of the psychological state of the mother that might be predictors of positive changes in the child's health at that time. Since morbidity at birth is often accounted for anomalies during gestation and childbirth, then the comparison of biological anamnesis of the mother and peculiarities of the child's health during the first years of living is of interest. Of course, not only the mother's health and diseases predetermine that change but they make their contribution to it. According to our

| The name of the diagnosis of the child made in the maternity ward | The first-year-old children | The second-year-old children |
|---|---|---|
| 1. Intrauterine hypoxia | 64 | 52 |
| 2. Physiological jaundice | 42 | 60 |
| 3. Conjugation jaundice | 4 | 6 |
| 4. Risk group due to perinatal encephalopathy | 15 | 8 |
| 5. Perinatal damage of central nervous system (CNS) | 4 | 6 |
| 6. Excitation syndrome | 2 | 2 |
| 7. Toxic erythema | 12 | 6 |
| 8. Hemorrhage in the skin | 12 | 20 |
| 9. Prematurity | 0 | 2 |
| 10. Morphofunctional immaturity | 2 | 2 |
| 11. Edema syndrome | 2 | 2 |
| 12. Low birth weight | 2 | 6 |
| 13. Large child | 8 | 6 |
| 14. Asphyxia of low level | 4 | 4 |
| 15. Asphyxia of mean level | 4 | 0 |
| 16. Asphyxia of high level | 2 | 0 |
| 17. Intrauterine growth restriction by hypotrophic type | 4 | 2 |
| 18. Cardiopathy | 4 | 2 |
| 19. Pathological loss of body weight | 2 | 8 |
| 20. Umbilical hernia | 0 | 2 |
| 21. Chin tremor | 0 | 2 |
| 22. Low muscle tones | 0 | 2 |
| 23. Muscle hypertonus | 0 | 2 |
| 24. Respiratory distress syndrome of type 1 | 0 | 2 |
| 25. Hypoxic damage of CNS | 0 | 2 |
| 26. The syndrome of CNS depression | 0 | 2 |
| 27. Oxygen-dependent child | 0 | 2 |
| 28. Depressed reflexes | 0 | 2 |
| 29. Mammary glands engorgement | 0 | 4 |
| 30. Right parietal cephalohematoma | 0 | 4 |
| 31. Perinatal contact with chronic hepatitis C virus | 2 | 2 |
| 32. Umbilical cord entanglement around the neck | 2 | 2 |
| 33. Nappy rash | 0 | 2 |
| 34. Hyperbilirubinemia | 0 | 2 |
| 35. The right-side dacryocystitis | 0 | 2 |
| 36. The left-side dacryocystitis | 0 | 2 |
| 37. The left-side flat valgus foot | 2 | 2 |
| 38. Reduced film of the tear duct | 0 | 4 |
| 39. Papilloma of the left areola | 2 | 0 |
| 40. Urinary tract infection | 2 | 0 |

| The name of the diagnosis of the child made in the maternity ward | The first-year-old children | The second-year-old children |
|---|---|---|
| 41. Ankyloglossia | 2 | 0 |
| 42. The right clavicle fracture | 2 | 0 |
| 43. Polycythemia | 2 | 0 |
| 44. Intrauterine hypotrophy | 2 | 0 |

**Table 2.**
*The children's diagnoses made in the maternity hospital (%).*

| The name of the diagnosis of the child made by local doctor | The ratio of the canceled and non-canceled diagnoses of children | | | | | |
|---|---|---|---|---|---|---|
| | The first-year-old | | | The second-year-old | | |
| | Number of diagnoses | Canceled | Non-canceled | Number of diagnoses | Cancelled | Non-canceled |
| Perinatal encephalopathy | 86 | 24 | 62 | 80 | 64 | 16 |
| Moving disorders | 54 | 20 | 34 | 48 | 36 | 12 |
| Excitation syndrome | 6 | 2 | 4 | 8 | 4 | 4 |
| Anemia | 2 | 0 | 2 | 4 | 0 | 4 |
| Atopic dermatitis | 4 | 2 | 2 | 4 | 0 | 4 |
| Flat valgus foot | 2 | 0 | 2 | 0 | 0 | 0 |
| Pyelectasis | 2 | 0 | 2 | 0 | 0 | 0 |
| Dysplasia of the hip joints | 2 | 0 | 2 | 0 | 0 | 0 |
| Hypotrophy of the 1,2,3 degrees | 0 | 0 | 0 | 6 | 6 | 0 |
| Inguinal hernia | 0 | 0 | 0 | 4 | 0 | 4 |
| Paratrophy | 2 | 2 | 0 | 2 | 0 | 2 |
| Cardiopathy | 2 | 0 | 2 | 0 | 0 | 0 |
| Little anomaly of heart development | 0 | 0 | 0 | 2 | 0 | 2 |

**Table 3.**
*The ratio of the canceled and non-canceled diagnoses for each of the diseases made by a local doctor.*

data, the mothers of the first- and second-year-old children do not differ between one another in the parameters of biological anamnesis.

Further, we have fulfilled correlation analysis (the Spearman's coefficient) aiming to identify relations between the children's health parameters and parameters of biological anamnesis of the mothers. There is a positive connection between the number of the diagnoses in the first- and second-year-old children during their stay in the maternity ward and perinatal pathology factors of the mother ($r = 0.336$, $p \leq 0.001$ for the first-year-old children; $r = 0.226$, $p \leq 0.05$ for the second-year-old children). Besides, the interrelation between the number of perinatal pathology factors and health group of the first- and second-year-old children is observed ($r = 0.243$, $p \leq 0.02$ for the first-year-old children; $r = 0.281$, $p \leq 0.01$ for the second-year-old children). There is no significant interrelation between the number of the diagnoses in the second-year-old children and perinatal pathology factors of their mothers. That is connected with that a part of diagnoses has been canceled by the moment of the examination of the child. However, the number of the diagnoses in the first-year-old children made by a local doctor is validly connected ($r = 0.478$, $p \leq 0.001$) with the quantity of perinatal pathology factors identified during their mothers' pregnancy.

There is a positive interrelation between the health group type of the second-year-old children and the presence of abortions made before by their mothers ($r = 0.213$, $p \leq 0.05$). One should point out that no similar relation is found in the first-year-old children. The obtained data evidence a negative effect of abortions on the children's health. It manifests and is detected after some time only. The results obtained in correlation analysis correspond to the results of single-factor analysis of variance. It has shown that exactly the number of the perinatal pathology factors of the mother influences the number of the children's diagnoses made in the maternity hospital (where $F = 9.565$, $p = 0.003$ for the first-year-old children; $F = 5.014$, $p = 0.030$ for the second-year-old children).

We have analyzed 28 parameters indicating the presence of pathology in the mother. Based on them, the control of the state of health and prevention of abnormalities are performed in the children who have risks of getting central nervous system disorders at the maternity house. The analysis reveals that only 8% of the mothers of first-year-old children and 14% of the second-year-old children are almost healthy. About 74 and 62% of the mothers have different extragenital diseases. The obstetric anamneses of 24% of the mothers, having first-year-old children, are burdened with abortions, 22% of the mothers—having second-year-old children. The anamneses of 8 and 10% of the women correspondingly are burden with miscarriage. The current pregnancy of 34% of the mothers of first-year-old children and 22% of the mothers of second-year-old children is complicated by the threat of abortion. In 18 and 10% of the mothers of children aged under 2 years old, it is accompanied by placental insufficiency. In 14% of the women, there is an immunological incompatibility of blood of the mother and the fetus. Besides, 6% of the women having first-year-old children and 2% of the women having second-year-old children have got the symptoms of fetal hypoxia. About 14% of the mothers of first-year-old children and 10% of the mothers of second-year-old children are characterized by weakness of labor. The dominant factors in the structure of extragenital anomalies of the mothers of first- and second-year-old children (as in some other investigations) are iron deficiency anemia (26%), kidney diseases (28 and 30%) and vegetovascular dystonia (24 and 20%).

In our further analysis, all the factors are divided into three groups according to the period of impact:

1. Detrimental factors during the progenesis.

2. Adverse factors during the antenatal period.

3. Adverse factors during the birth period (the intranatal period).

We cannot detect any role of factors in progenesis, since we have observed the women regarding the gestation responsibly and regularly consulting with a gynecologist during their pregnancy. Only 4% of the mothers of first-year-old children smoke; and among the mothers of second-year-old children, there are no women with bad habits. About 4% of the mothers of children aged under one-year-old and 12% of the mothers of second-year-old children have gynecological diseases in the anamnesis.

But we have been able to show the influence of the factors of perinatal pathology in the mother during the antenatal period on the future health of the child. The most significant factors of risk of the child's morbidity are the following: the threat of abortion (34% of the first-year-old children's mothers and 22% of the second-year-old children's mothers), anemia (26%), vegetovascular dystonia (24 and 20%), kidney diseases (28 and 30%) and chronic fetoplacental insufficiency (18 and 10%). During the intranatal period, the significant risk factors of perinatal pathology of the mothers, exerting influence upon the health of the first- and second-year-old children, are episiotomy (20 and 26%), cesarean (26 and 16%), premature rupture of membranes (20 and 18%) and weakness of labor activity (14 and 10%). We have not found any substantial differences in the pathology of the mothers of two groups. But this distribution shows the typical situation for pregnant women in Russia [25].

Correlation analysis of the results about the interrelation of the number of diagnoses in the first-year-old children, made by a local doctor, with perinatal anomaly factors during the antenatal period is in **Table 4**. We have found the significant relation of the children's morbidity with fetoplacental insufficiency during pregnancy ($r = 0.444$, $p < 0.001$) as well as with threat of abortion ($r = 0.379$, $p < 0.01$) and gestosis in the mother during pregnancy ($r = 0.353$, $p < 0.01$). We have revealed the close positive relation between the first-year-old children's health deterioration and iron deficiency anemia ($r = 0.330$, $p < 0.02$) and kidney diseases ($r = 0.276$, $p < 0.05$) through the mother. That is, the more diseases the mother has, the higher number of diseases the first-year-old children have.

There is no significant correlation relationship between the number of diseases of the second-year-old children and perinatal pathology factors of the mother during the antenatal period. However, significant interconnection is found between the number of diseases of the second-year-old children and iron efficiency anemia ($r = 0.382$, $p < 0.01$), varicosity ($r = 0.332$, $p < 0.02$), and the mother's kidney diseases ($r = 0.281$, $p < 0.05$). The analysis of the results about the interrelation of the number of diagnoses in the first-year-old children (by a local doctor) with the perinatal pathology factors of the mother during the intranatal period is in **Table 5**. It has revealed the significance of that dependence with weakness of birth activity ($r = 0.354$, $p < 0.001$). There is no similar association in the second-year-old children.

| Mother's perinatal pathology | The number of diagnoses, made by a local doctor | |
|---|---|---|
| | The first-year-old children | The second-year-old children |
| Fetoplacental insufficiency | r = 0.444, p < 0.001 | p > 0.05 |
| Threat of abortion | r = 0.379, p < 0.01 | p > 0.05 |
| Gestosis | r = 0.353, p < 0.01 | p > 0.05 |
| Iron efficiency anemia | r = 0.330, p < 0.02 | r = 0.382, p < 0.01 |
| Kidney diseases | r = 0.276, p < 0.05 | r = 0,281, p < 0.05 |
| Varicosity | p > 0.05 | r = 0.322, p < 0.02 |

**Table 4.**
*Correlations between the number of diagnosis and factors of the mother's perinatal pathology.*

We have revealed (**Table 5**) close interrelation between the number of diagnoses, made by a local doctor, and premature childbirth of the mother ($r = 0.663$, $p < 0.001$) for the second-year-old children.

One might suppose that the degree of influence of those factors upon children of different sex would be different (**Table 6**). We have found close positive interconnection between the number of the first-year-old girls' diagnoses and their mothers' diseases of the cardiovascular system ($r = 0.581$, $p < 0.01$), iron deficiency anemia and kidney diseases ($r = 0.529$, $p < 0.02$; $r = 0.463$, $p < 0.05$) as well as fetoplacental insufficiency ($r = 0.489$, $p < 0.05$). As for the boys, there is a positive relationship between the number of diagnoses and gestosis in the mother during pregnancy ($r = 0.400$, $p < 0.001$), the threat of premature childbirth ($r = 0.374$, $p < 0.05$), immunological incompatibility of blood of the mother and the fetus ($r = 0.457$, $p < 0.01$) and kidney diseases ($r = 0.391$, $p < 0.01$).

The analysis of the results about the relationship of the number of diagnoses in the second-year-old girls with the perinatal pathology factors during the antenatal period reveals significant dependence between the child's morbidity and iron deficiency anemia and edema in the mother during pregnancy ($r = 0.509$, $p < 0.02$; $r = 0.780$, $p < 0.001$ correspondingly). It is noteworthy that close relationship is found between the number of diseases in the second-year-old boys and kidney diseases in the mother ($r = 0.484$, $p < 0.01$). Besides, significant positive relation is identified between the number of diseases in the second-year-old boys and negative Rh factor of the mother ($r = 0,508$, $p < 0.001$), and iron deficiency anemia ($r = 0.494$, $p < 0.01$).

The result of correlation analysis between the antenatal pathology factors of the mother and the number of diagnoses, made by a local doctor separately for the boys and girls, are in **Table 6**.

Further, we carry out correlation analysis aimed at identifying the interrelation of the number of diagnoses in the boys and girls, made by a local doctor, with the perinatal anomaly factors during the intranatal period (**Table 7**).

Close positive connection reveals between the number of diagnoses in the first-year-old girls, made by a local doctor, and episiotomy ($r = 0.552$, $p < 0.01$), and premature rupture of membranes in the mother ($r = 0.586$, $p < 0.01$). There is association between the number of diagnoses of the first-year-old boys and weakness of labor activity of the mother ($r = 0.457$, $p < 0.01$).

The analysis of the results about the interconnection between the number of diagnoses in the second-year-old girls and the perinatal pathology factors during delivery reveals significant dependence, the defect of the placenta ($r = 0.780$, $p < 0.001$) and manual control of the uterine cavity at childbirth ($r = 0.453$, $p < 0.05$). There is no significance of the same associations in the second-year-old boys. Subsequently, the health of children aged under 2 years old changes significantly during the first 2 years of life. The less factors of perinatal anomalies the

| **Pathology factors of the mother during the intranatal period** | **The number of diagnoses of children** | |
|---|---|---|
| | **The first-year-old children** | **The second-year-old children** |
| weakness of birth activity | $r = 0.354$, $p < 0.01$ | $p > 0.05$ |
| premature childbirth | $p > 0.05$ | $r = 0.633$, $p < 0.001$ |

**Table 5.**
*The interrelation of the number of diagnoses of children (by a local doctor) with the perinatal pathology factors of the mother during the intranatal period.*

| **The antenatal pathology factors of the mother** | **The number of diagnoses made by a local doctor** | | | |
|---|---|---|---|---|
| Number of diagnoses of boys and girls (by a local doctor) | **The first-year-old children** | | **The second-year-old-children** | |
| | **Girls** | **Boys** | **Girls** | **Boys** |
| Fetoplacental insufficiency | r = 0.489, p < 0.05 | p > 0.05 | p > 0.05 | p > 0.05 |
| Gestosis | p > 0.05 | r = 0.400, p < 0,001 | p > 0.05 | p > 0.05 |
| The threat of premature childbirth | p > 0.05 | r = 0.374, p < 0.05 | p > 0.05 | p > 0.05 |
| Diseases of the cardiovascular system | r = 0.581, p < 0.01 | p > 0.05 | p > 0.05 | p > 0.05 |
| Iron deficiency anemia | r = 0.529, p < 0.02 | p > 0.05 | r = 0.509, p < 0.02 | r = 0.494, p < 0.01 |
| Kidney diseases | r = 0.463, p < 0.05 | r = 0.391, p < 0.01 | p > 0.05 | r = 0.484, p < 0.01 |
| Immunological incompatibility of blood | p > 0.05 | r = 0.457, p < 0.01 | p > 0.05 | r = 0.508, p < 0.001 |
| Edema | p > 0.05 | p > 0.05 | r = 0.780, p < 0.001 | p > 0.05 |

**Table 6.**
*The interrelation of the number of diagnoses of boys and girls (by a local doctor) with the perinatal pathology factors of the mother during the antenatal period.*

| **The intranatal pathology factors of the mother** | **Of the number of diagnoses made by a local doctor** | | | |
|---|---|---|---|---|
| | **The first-year-old children** | | **The second-year-old children** | |
| | **Girls** | **Boys** | **Girls** | **Boys** |
| Episiotomy | r = 0.552, p < 0.01 | p > 0.05 | p > 0.05 | p > 0.05 |
| premature rupture of membranes | r = 0.586, p < 0.01 | p > 0.05 | p > 0.05 | p > 0.05 |
| weakness of labor activity | p > 0.05 | r = 0.457, p < 0.01 | p > 0.05 | p > 0.05 |
| the defect of the placenta | p > 0.05 | p > 0.05 | r = 0.780, <0.001 | p > 0.05 |
| manual control of the uterine cavity | p > 0.05 | p > 0.05 | r = 0.453, p < 0.05 | p > 0.05 |

**Table 7.**
*The interrelation of the number of diagnoses of boys and girls (by a local doctor) with the perinatal pathology factors of the mother during the intranatal period.*

mother has got, the more positive prognosis with regard to the child's health is. The most widespread diagnoses of the child at birth are encephalopathy and syndrome of motor disorders. The leading groups of the factors of perinatal pathology of the mother are extragenital diseases and birth activity complications. The change of the relationship between the number of diagnoses of the children at the age of the first 2 years old and the perinatal pathology factors of the mother is different in the boys and girls.

Maternal pathology leads to low level of oxygen during pregnancy and followed the different child disorders [46].

### 3.3 The influence of psychological features of the mother on the child's health

It is obvious that not only perinatal pathology contributes to the health of the child at an early age [46]. Moreover, the success of child care during the first years of life is determined by psychological features of the mother. And that is why we will address the assessment of the influence of emotional reaction of the mother to the child's health status. Univariate analysis of variance is carried out to evaluate the influence of independent variable "the degree of the mother's attachment to the child" [47, 48] on the future possible cancelation of the child's diagnosis by a local doctor. The significant influence is obtained for one scale of the questionnaire only. Based on the results of the research, the degree of acceptance of the child (the acceptance-rejection scale) by the mothers of first-year-old children exerts influence on the probability of cancelation of the child's diagnosis made by a local pediatrician ($F = 6.829$, $p < 0.003$) during the first 2 years.

There are no differences between the mothers of first- and second-year-old children according to the degrees of attachment. About 54% of the mothers of each group are characterized by low degree of attachment; 44 and 42% correspondingly are characterized by mean degree. Only 2 and 4% of the mothers of first- and second-year-old children have high degree of attachment. No mothers with maternal deprivation are identified. Positive prognosis in terms of health of the first-year-old children depends upon the degree of acceptance of the child by the mother: the higher the value on the acceptance-rejection scale is, the better the child's health is. Our data point to the absence of differences in the features of emotional intelligence of the mothers of the first- and second-year-old children. The similarity of emotional intelligence of the mothers is explained by that they represent the same social environment.

The research results show that the majority of the mothers are characterized by low level of the capability to understand and control their own and other emotions as well as of interpersonal, intrapersonal and general emotional intelligence. There are no mothers with high level of emotional intelligence. Probably, that is why we do not find any association between emotional intelligence of the mother and the probability of cancelation of the child's diagnosis either in variance or correlation analysis. At the same time, in a sample of the mothers of second-year-old children, univariate analysis of variance reveals the influence of independent variables "understanding of other emotions" and "general emotional intelligence" on dependent variable "degree of attachment" ($F = 2.115$, $p = 0.051$; $F = 2.618$, $p = 0.029$). The better the understanding of other emotions and general emotional intelligence are, the higher the degree of attachment is. We have detected the influence of independent variables "understanding of other emotions", "control of expression" and "control of one's own and other emotions" on dependent variable "sensitivity-insensitivity" (correspondingly, $F = 3.741$, $p = 0.002$; $F = 3.714$, $p = 0.003$; $F = 2.747$, $p = 0.015$). The higher the values of the structural components of emotional intelligence are, the more efficient the mother is. That is, she respects for the child's independency to a greater extent.

Our data refer only to those women who led predominantly healthy lives before pregnancy and actively cared for the child immediately after his (her) birth. It is consistent with a large number of studies showing the dependence of the health level of the child at birth on both the mother's health before pregnancy and her pathology that arose during pregnancy and during childbirth [1, 7, 18, 19]. Our data show that the acceptance of the child is the main psychological factor that contributes to the recovery of the child by the end of the second year his (her) life. At the same time, there are no significant effects between the parameters of emotional intelligence and the child's recovery. Although the parameters of emotional intelligence affect the sensitivity of the mother to the child needs. Perhaps in another sample, in which mothers with high level of the emotional intelligence would participate, such connections will be found.

## 4. Conclusions

Almost all the children at birth have one or the other diagnosis (96% of the first- and second-year-old children). But by the end of the first year of life, diagnoses are canceled in 40% of the children by a local doctor, and during the second year of life—in 60% of the children. The most widespread diagnose of the child at birth is perinatal encephalopathy and syndrome of motor disorders.

Only 8% of the first-year-old children's mothers and 14% of the second-year-old children's mothers are almost healthy. The less factors of perinatal pathology there are in the mother, the more positive the prognosis with regard to the child's health within the first 2 years of living is. The association of morbidity of the children with the factors of perinatal pathology of the mother is the most pronounced during the first year of living. During the second year of life, the boys' health is less dependent on those factors than that of the girls.

There are differences between the mothers of first- and second-year-old children according to the degrees of attachment. About 54% of the mothers of each group are characterized by low degree of attachment; 44 and 42% correspondingly are characterized by mean degree. Only 2 and 4% of the mothers of the first- and second-year-old children are characterized by high degree of attachment. No mothers with maternal deprivation have been identified. Positive prognosis with regard to the first-year-old children's health depends upon the acceptance of the child by the mother: the higher the value on the scale of acceptance-nonacceptance is, the better the child's health is.

The degree of emotional intelligence of the mother is not associated with the probability of cancelation of the child's diagnosis.

## Acknowledgements

The work was supported by the grant of the Russian Fund of the Fundamental Researches# 18-413-480007.

## Conflict of interest

We have no any conflict of interest.

**Author details**

Elena Nikolaeva[1,2*] and Vera Merenkova[2]

1 Herzen State Pedagogical University, Saint-Petersburg, Russian Federation

2 Bunin Yelets State University, Yelets, Russian Federation

*Address all correspondence to: klemtina@yandex.ru

## References

[1] Aboud FE, Yousafzai AK. Global health and development in early childhood. Annual Review of Psychology. 2015;**66**:433-457

[2] Vergunov EG, Nikolaeva EI, Balioz NV, Krivoschekov SG. Lateral preferences as the possible phenotypic predictors of the reserves of the cardiovascular system and the features of sensorimotor integration in climbers. Human Physiology. 2018;**44**(3):12-21

[3] Gage SH, Munaf MR, Smith GD. Causal inference in developmental origins of health and disease (DOHaD) research. Annual Review of Psychology. 2016;**67**:567-585

[4] Rancour-Laferriere D. The Slave Soul of Russia: Moral Masochism and the Cult of Suffering. New York: New York University Press; 1996

[5] Nikolaeva EI, Merenkova VS. The effect of a Mother's level of attachment and her emotional intelligence on a child's health during its first year of life. Psychology. 2013;**4**(5):483-487

[6] Honigfeld LS, Kaplan DW. Native American post neonatal mortality. Pediatrics. 1987;**80**(4):575-578

[7] Amorim D, Machadom HS. Newborn and maternal outcomes in out-of-hospital delivery: A review. Journal of Pregnancy and Child Health. 2018;**5**(2). DOI: 10.4172/2376-127X.1000371

[8] Cohain JS. Apgar score of 0 at 5 min and neonatal seizures or serious neurologic dysfunction in relation to birth setting. American Journal of Obstetrics and Gynecology. 2014;**210**:377

[9] Lai MC, Yang SN. Perinatal hypoxic-ischemic encephalopathy. Journal of Biomedicine & Biotechnology. 2011:609-813

[10] Northington FJ, Chavez-Valdez R, Martin LJ. Neuronal cell death in neonatal hypoxia-ischemia. Annals of Neurology. 2011;**69**:743-758

[11] Velimirsky M, Sak P. Management of pregnancy with premature rupture of membranes (prom). Journal of Health Sciences Management and Public Health. 2004;**59**(9):669-677. DOI: 10.1097/01.ogx.0000137610.33201.a4

[12] Repina MA. Gestosis as a cause of maternal mortality. Obstetric and Women's Diseases. 2000;**XLIX**(3):11-18

[13] Hanson MA, Gluckman PD. Developmental origins of health and disease: New insights. Basic & Clinical Pharmacology & Toxicology. 2008;**102**:90-93

[14] Distefano G, Pratico AD. Actualities on molecular pathogenesis and repairing process of cerebral damage in perinatal hypoxic-ischemic encephalopathy. Italian Journal of Pediatrics. 2010;**36**:63

[15] Ray-Santano C, Mielgo VE, Gastiasoro E, Murgia X, Lafuente H, Ruix-del-Yerro E, et al. Early cerebral hemodynamic, metabolic, and histological changes in hypoxic-ischemic fetal lambs during postnatal life. Frontiers in Neuroscience. 2011;**5**:111

[16] Duda VI. Ostetrics. Textbook. M: Visheishaja shkola; 2002

[17] Erick M. Hyperemesis gravidarum: A case of starvation and altered sensorium gestosis (ASG). Medical Hypotheses. 2014;**82**(5):572-580 https://doi.org/10.1016/j.mehy.2014.02.014

[18] Avramenko NV, Kabachenko OV, Barkovsky DE, Mykhailenko MO, Shkrobotko NV. Risk factors delivery of

the newborns with distress. Zaporožskij Medicinskij Žurnal. 2014;(2):62-63. DOI: 10.14739/2310-1210.2014.2.25427

[19] Aziz N, Cheng YV, Caugey AB. Neonatal outcomes in the setting of preterm premature rupture of membranes complicated by chorioamnionitis. The Journal of Maternal-Fetal & Neonatal Medicine. 2009;**22**(9):780-784

[20] Cousens S, Blencowe H, Gravett M, Lawn JE. Antibiotics for pre-term pre-labour rupture of membranes: Prevention of neonatal deaths due to complications of pre-term birth and infection. International Journal of Epidemiology. 2010;**39**(Suppl 1): 134-143

[21] Cobo T, Palacio M, Martinez-Terron M, Navarro-Sastre A, Bosch J, Filella X, et al. Clinical and inflammatory markers in amniotic fluid as predictors of adverse outcomes in preterm premature rupture of membranes. American Journal of Obstetrics and Gynecology. 2011;**205**(2):126.e1-126.e8

[22] Erdemer G, Kultursay N, Calcavur S, Zekioglu O, Koroglu OA, Cakmak B, et al. Histological chorioamnionitis: Effects on premature delivery and neonatal prognosis. Pediatrics And Neonatology. 2013;**54**(4):267-274

[23] Harrison MS, Goldenberg RL. Global burden of prematurity. Seminars in Fetal & Neonatal Medicine. 2016;**21**(2):74-79

[24] Menton R, Taylir RN, Fortunato SJ. Chorioamnionitis – A complex pathophysiologic syndrome. Placenta. 2010;**31**(2):113-120

[25] Oxenoit GK, Nikitina CY, Ageev LI, Aleksandrova GA, Zaichenko NM, Kirillov GN, et al. Zdravoohranenije in Russia. M. Rosstat; 2017

[26] Nikolaeva EI, Merenkova VS. Psychological and psychophysiological mechanisms of influence of child care quality on his health. Voprosi psychologii. 2015;**36**(3):52-59

[27] Nikolaeva EI, Merenkova VS. The influence of the mother's attachment to the child of the first years of life and her response to the emotional situation on the child's health. Voprosi psychologii. 2010;**2**:65-72

[28] Nikolaeva EI. Alexander Luria: Creator in the perspective of time. Cognitive Systems Monographs. 2015;**25**:457-468

[29] Bowlby J. Maternal Care and Mental Health. The Master Work Series. 2nd ed. Northvale, NJ; London: Jason Aronson; 1995. ISBN 1-56821-757-9. OCLC 33105354. [Geneva, World Health Organization, Monograph series no. 3, 1950]

[30] Oteva EA, Nikolaeva EI, NIkolaeva AA, Sartakova BN, Parm YN. Assessment of the health status of pregnant women in Novosibirsk scientific center: Somatic and psychological aspects. Obstetrics and Gynecology. 1994;**3**:25-27

[31] Bowlby J. Attachment and Loss. Vol. 3: Loss, Sadness and Depression. New York: Basic Books; 1980

[32] Bowlby J. A Secure Base: Parent-Child Attachment and Healthy Human Development. Tavistock Professional Book. London: Routledge; 1988. ISBN 0-422-62230-3. OCLC 42913724

[33] Ainsworth MD, Blehar M, Waters E, Wall S. Patterns of Attachment: A Psychological Study of the Strange Situation. Hillsdale, NJ: Lawrence Erlbaum; 1978

[34] Crittenden P. Danger and development: The organization of self-protective strategies. In: Vondra JI, Barnett D, editors. Atypical Attachment in Infancy and Early Childhood among

Children at Developmental Risk. Oxford: Blackwell; 1999. pp. 145-171

[35] Bar-On R. The Bar-on Emotional Quotient Inventory (EQ-I): Technical Manual. Toronto: Multi-Health Systems; 1997

[36] Bradberry T, Greaves J. The Emotional Intelligence Quick Book. New York: Simon and Schuster; 2005

[37] Caruso DR, Mayer JD, Salovey P. Relation of an ability measure of emotional intelligence to personality. Journal of Personality Assessment. 2002;**79**:306-320

[38] Mayer JD, Salovey P, Caruso DR, Sitarenios G. Emotional intelligence as a standard intelligence. Emotion. 2001;**1**:232-242

[39] Booth-Laforce C, Oh W, Kim AH, Rubin KH, Rose-Krasnor L, Burgess K. Attachment, self-worth, and peer-group functioning in middle childhood. Attachment & Human Development. 2006;**8**(4):309-325

[40] Vygotsky LS. Mind in society: The development of higher psychological processes. In: Cole M, John-Steiner V, Scribner S, Souberman E, editors. Cambridge, Massachusetts: Harvard University Press; 1978

[41] Nikolaeva EI, Merenkova VS. An inner picture of health as a factor in changing a child's behavior to health-promoting behavior. Psychology in Russia: State of the Art. 2017;**10**(4):162-171

[42] Sheeran P, Klein WMP, Rothman AJ. Health behavior change: Moving from observation to intervention. Annual Review of Psychology. 2017;**68**:573-600

[43] Liusin DV. New technique for measuring emotional intelligence: EmIn's questionnaire. Psychological Diagnostics. 2006;**4**:3-22

[44] Helgeson VC, Zajdel M. Adjusting to chronic health conditions. Annual Review of Psychology. 2017;**68**:545-571

[45] Shah PS, Perlman M. Time courses of intrapartum asphyxia: Neonatal characteristics and outcomes. American Journal of Perinatology. 2009;**26**:39-44

[46] Friedman HS, Kern ML. Personality, well-being, and health. Annual Review of Psychology. 2014;**65**:719-742

[47] Perlman JM. The genesis of cognitive and behavioral deficits in premature graduates of intensive care. Minerva Pediatrica. 2003;**55**(2):89-101

[48] Vereshagina NV, Nikolaeva EI. Test questionnaire assessing the mother's attitude to the child of the first two years of life. Voprosi psychologii. 2009;**4**:151-159

Chapter 2

# Public Policies for Promotion of Maternal-Infant Health in Brazil: Some Experiences with Adolescent Mothers in São Paulo

*Aline Mizutani Gomes and Renato Alves*

## Abstract

This chapter introduces and discusses to what extent policies focused on promoting maternal and infant health through public health services are or are not effective in the coverage area. The discussion is based on accounts of adolescents—mothers or still pregnant—and the assistance provided to them and their children through these services. The accounts, which are derived from an independent program of home visits to accompany these adolescents, are complemented by observations made by the visitation team about whether assistance provided by health services promote maternal and infant health and the rights of children and adolescents. To provide context, we present a panorama of current public-health policies and services aimed at mothers and infants in Brazil, as well as some health indicators for this population. Finally, we discuss the possibilities and challenges of promoting the healthy development of mothers and their children in these contexts.

**Keywords:** public policies, promotion of maternal-infant health, adolescent pregnancy, prenatal, maternal-infant mortality

## 1. Introduction

Brazil is a country of continental dimensions, with enormous geographic and cultural diversity and with major problems of social inequality. To get an idea of the regional differences, while the north region is covered by the Amazon rainforest, has the largest population that self-identifies as indigenous, and accounts for 42.25% of Brazil's territory with the lowest population density, the southeast region is the most populous, has the largest urban center, greatest industrial output, and accounts for more than 50% of everything the country produces (in GDP terms) [1].

Furthermore, in the past decade, the country has undergone both advances and setbacks, in terms of politics and economics, that have directly influenced the development of its public policies, including those in regard to maternal-infant health, the focus of this chapter. In this sense, although currently there are important investments in programs focused on reducing maternal-infant mortality rates, humanizing services, and promoting the healthy development of the population, the country still has a long way to go.

In historic terms, the passage of the 1988 Constitution was an important step in the process of changing the paradigm of Brazilian health policies, in that it began to address the concept of health as a right of all citizens and the obligation of the state. This prioritization led to the creation of the Unified Health System (Sistema Único de Saúde or SUS), which is geared toward providing free services to all individuals, ranging from the simplest outpatient consultations to more complex surgeries, and which represents one of the largest public health systems in the world, offering integrated, universal, and egalitarian access to all Brazilian citizens [2, 3].

SUS promotes the regionalization of services; hierarchization into increasingly complex levels, depending on the needs of the population being served; the decentralization of command, giving autonomy to each sphere of power to make its decisions; and the participation of the population in the system's day-to-day operations. All these principles seek not only to prevent illnesses but also work toward promoting health, quality of life, economic and social development, and the reduction of inequalities [4].

Also worth mentioning is the Child and Adolescent Statute (Estatuto da Criança e do Adolescente or ECA) of 1990, which includes eight articles dedicated to rights to life and health. This statute has been praised for the advances it provides in the form that children and adolescents are viewed in the country. As a result, it seeks to ensure dignified conditions of life, starting even before birth, considering that articles 7 and 8 guarantee that pregnant mothers and newborns have access to pre- and perinatal services by way of public policies that promote healthy development [5].

Also included in the social advances relevant to the promotion of health and improved quality of life of the population—especially mothers and children—we should note the role of the Bolsa Familia Program. Created in 2003, this is a wealth-transfer program at the federal level that helps families living in poverty and extreme poverty to break the intergenerational cycle of poverty. Furthermore, it seeks to contribute to the expansion of access to public services that represent basic rights in the areas of health, education, and social assistance, representing one of the main factors that have led to the reduction in infant mortality [6].

## 2. Brief overview of maternal-infant health policies

As noted above, the Brazilian health system is organized around the SUS, for which financing is carried out through resources raised from taxes and social contributions, and which is managed at the national level by the Health Ministry. The ministry is also responsible for creating and monitoring policies and activities that are implemented according to the needs of municipal managers, in accordance with the principle of decentralization [2, 8].

Among the main structural policies of the SUS, we highlight the Family Health Strategy (ESF), a program used to structure basic services—that is, the first level of health services and the population's entryway for receiving services through the system. The main characteristic of the ESF is the establishment of a team of various professionals—composed of general practitioners or specialists in family health, a nurse practitioner or specialist in family health, nursing assistant or technician, and community health agents (ACSs)—and the establishment of a territory for them to cover, thereby complying with the principle of regionalization of the SUS. As a result, the unique aspect of this program is that it allows the health team to become acquainted with the local reality and the needs of the population, establishing links between the team and users, which in turn increases the adoption of treatments and interventions proposed by the health professionals [7, 8].

The ESF health team is linked to the local Basic Health Unit (UBS). At the UBS, Brazilians can receive free basic treatment in pediatrics, gynecology, general medicine, nursing, and odontology. The main services offered are medical consultations, inhalations, injections, dressing of wounds, vaccines, collection for laboratory exams, odontological treatment, referrals to specialists, and the provision of basic medications. Generally, the UBS is located close to the user's home, and it is there that services are carried out for prenatal, post-natal, and infant care [7, 8].

Under the *National Policy of Basic Services* [7], it was determined that each UBS should serve at most 12,000 inhabitants in large urban centers, with a maximum of 750 people per ACS, and 12 ACSs per Family Health team. Each Family Health team should be responsible for at most 4000 people, with the recommendation being an average of 3000 people. These limits are important in order to ensure quality service, especially under the logic of the ESF, which prioritizes ties with the population.

Among the specific policies of maternal-infant health, the first we will highlight is the *National Policy for Integrated Women's Health Services* [9], which:

> *"incorporates, with a gender focus, a holistic approach and the promotion of health as its guiding principles, and seeks to consolidate advances in the field of sexual and reproductive rights, with an emphasis on improved obstetric services, family planning, attention to unsafe abortions, and combating domestic and sexual violence."*

This policy was an update of the 1983 *Program of Integrated Women's Health Services* (PAISM), which was an important step in Brazilian women's mobilization to defend their reproductive rights. Therefore, the National Policy for Integrated Women's Health Services represents an advance in terms of integrating women's health services, with special attention to family planning, educational activities to prevent undesired pregnancies and sexually transmitted diseases, and in terms of encouraging corporal autonomy [9].

Even with these advances in the attention given to women's health services, the impact on indicators was lower than expected. That is why, in 2000, the *Program for the Humanization of Birth and Pre-Natal Services* (PHPN) was implemented, with the main objective being the reduction in high rates of maternal, perinatal and neonatal, mortality through the provision of improved access, coverage, and quality of prenatal, birthing, and infant assistance. One of the initiatives of this program is the right of pregnant mothers to visit and create ties with the maternity ward where they will be served, and the guarantee that mothers can have a companion present during labor, delivery, and postpartum periods [10].

The issue of humanizing services has been shown to be directly related to the quality of services provided, and the capacity to make resolute and satisfactory decisions. This is not just a labeling matter, but one of creating a hospitable environment where rights are recognized, specific needs are respected, and knowledge is shared. One of the major impediments to carrying out any public policy is precisely in the passage from theory to practice. It is not enough to have a progressive discourse and innovative ideas if these are not based on concrete experiences, synchronizing the needs of the population with the proposed intervention [11].

In this sense, humanized prenatal and infant services imply a reorganization of the work processes, facilitating access to health services, and integrating new levels of attention. Furthermore, the policy provides new resources to pay for these services in order to assist most municipalities in implementing these activities according to the following criteria: carrying out the first prenatal consultation before the fourth month of pregnancy; guaranteeing at least six prenatal consultations, preferably with one coming in the first trimester, two in the second trimester, and three in the third trimester of pregnancy; one consultation up to 42 days after birth; lab exams such as (a) ABO-Rh during the first visit, (b) one Venereal Disease Research Laboratory during the first visit and another close to the thirtieth week of pregnancy, (c) routine urine tests, with one during the first visit and another close to the thirtieth week of pregnancy, (d) monitoring blood sugar levels, with one test during the first visit and another close to the thirtieth week of pregnancy, (e) hemoglobin/hematocrit exam during the first week, and offering to test for HIV, with one exam during the first visit in municipalities whose population is greater than 50,000; and applying tetanus vaccines up to the immunizing (second) dose or a reinforcement dose for women who have already been immunized [10].

In 2011, the Health Ministry created the *Stork Network*, a new program that sought to provide even more thorough women's health services at all stages of life, including actions geared toward assisting children up to 2 years of age. The structural concepts included range from respect for cultural, ethnic, and racial diversity; promotion of equity; focus on gender; expanding access to and improvement of prenatal care without unnecessary interventions; guaranteeing safe deliveries; and healthy development within the scope of the SUS. It also includes professional training as a strategy to achieve these improvements—after all, in addition to physical and technological facilities, services that seek to promote health in a holistic way depend on competent and sensitive professionals capable of taking a wider view than those circumscribed by biomedical aspects [12].

## 3. Pregnancy during adolescence

Between 2003 and 2016, on average, 6.6% of adolescents between 15 and 19 years of age became mothers. It is possible to note that during this period of time, the rate declined from 7.4% (2003) to 5.7% (2016). Despite this reduction, Brazilian rates are still very high when compared with the US and Canada. In 2015, rates for these countries stood at, respectively, 2.2% [13] and 1.1% [14].

The average rate of adolescent pregnancy in the city of São Paulo—the country's largest city—is a bit lower than the national average, coming in at 5.2% for the 2003–2016 period. However, somewhat differently than what happened nationally, the rate of pregnancy among adolescents remained relatively stable during this period, and showed signs of decline only starting in 2015 (**Figure 1**).

Pregnancy and motherhood during adolescence are topics that have been discussed a lot, the subject of analyses by different areas, and in general treated as a problem that creates difficulties not only for the adolescent mothers but also for their children and, at the end of the day, to society as a whole.

However, for a long time, the age range of 15–19 years was considered the ideal period for women to begin their reproductive lives. Among indigenous population, for example, teen pregnancy is viewed as natural. Furthermore, regional differences in terms of adolescent pregnancy is obvious, with pregnancy rates among 15–19-year olds in the north region of Brazil reaching 23.2%, while in the south, this rate is 13.8% (2016). Therefore, we can conclude that the notion of adolescent pregnancy being a problem reflects more the social, cultural, economic, and demographic issues of a community than biomedical risks. And as such, we cannot homogenize or generalize about the conceptions of what leads an adolescent woman to become pregnant [15–18].

According to Heilborn et al. [18], pregnancy during adolescence could be:

> *"[...] unexpected or the result of planning; could result in bonds, with subsequent separation; in more stable and lasting relationships; [...] it could result in irresponsible parenting or, to the contrary, turn out to be an antidote to anomie for adolescents [...] non-cohabitation, partial cohabitation, or dual residences."*

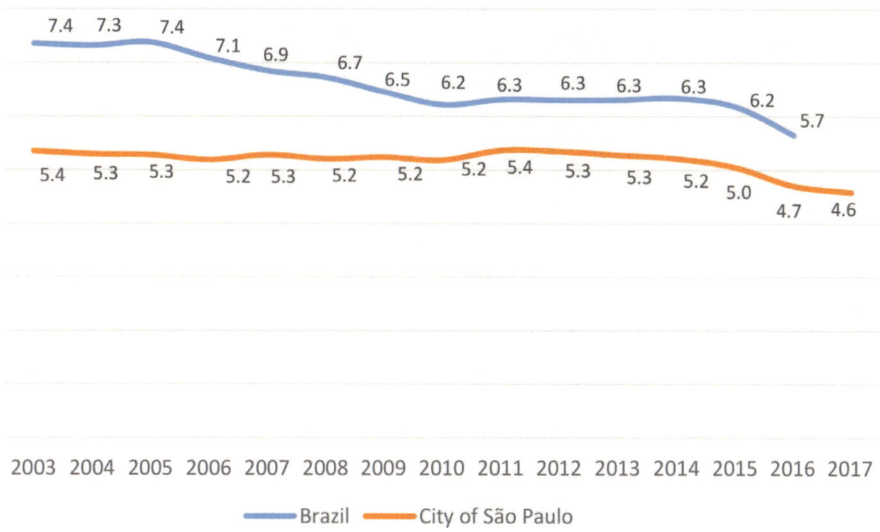


**Figure 1.**
*Proportion of pregnant adolescents between 15 and 19 years of age in Brazil and in the city of São Paulo. Source: DATASUS/TabNet/Municipal Health Department of the City of São Paulo [22].*

Another major point of debate is whether pregnancy during adolescence leads to an increase in school drop-out rates. However, Barbosa [19] showed that the rate of fertility among youths who are not in school is much higher than that for youths who are still in school. Based on this data, it seems that in reality, being out of school leads these youths to have no outlook other than the alternative of having children, and not the other way around.

Furthermore, there are significant differences in the educational trajectories of different social classes. While the experience of maternity among adolescents with higher incomes tends to only temporarily interrupt their school career—which for the most part is linear and generally resumed sometime after the birth of the child—among poorer classes, adolescent pregnancy proves to be much more harmful to the continuity of this trajectory, especially when there is an imperative need for the adolescent to reconcile mothering activities with some type of work that ensures the livelihood of the mother and her child [18].

Similar to what happens across the different regions of Brazil, in the city of São Paulo there is an inverse relationship between economic, social, and cultural conditions and adolescent pregnancy. To get an idea of the scale of this disparity, the average rate of adolescent pregnancy among the three wealthiest regions of the city is approximately 0.5%, whereas among the three poorest regions that rate is 7.5% (**Figure 2**). In other words, the chances of an adolescent from a poorer neighborhood getting pregnant are 16 times greater than for an adolescent in wealthier districts.

With regard to the biological risks of adolescent pregnancy, we should distinguish between pregnancy that occurs between the ages of 10 and 14 (which represents just 0.8% of cases) and pregnancies that occur between the ages of 15 and 19. Instances of restricted intrauterine growth, feto-pelvic disproportion, and retarded uterine development occur more frequently among girls between the ages of 10 and 14 years. We also note that situations of maternal or infant death, premature birth, low birth weight, gestational diabetes, anemia, and pre-eclampsia are much more closely related to precarious prenatal and birthing assistance than to the age at which pregnancy occurs [20, 21].

According to data from the Municipal Health Department, the number of weeks of pregnancy is not significantly different across various age groups. The majority

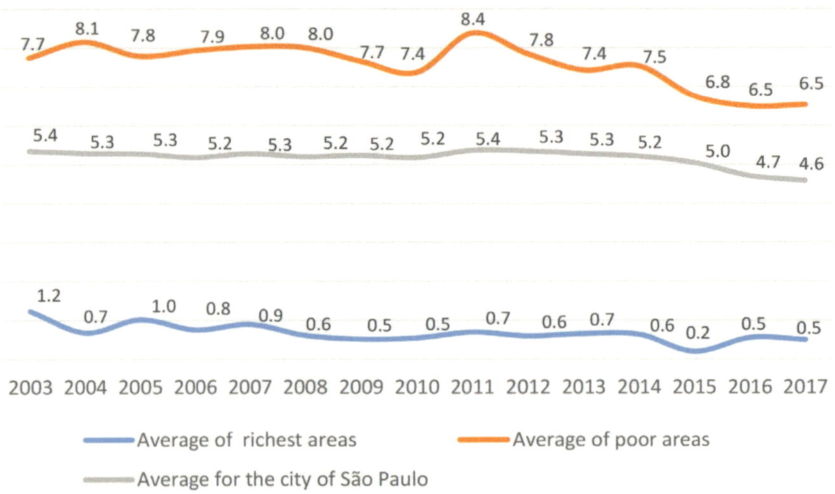


**Figure 2.**
*Comparison between average rates of adolescent pregnancy. Source: DATASUS/TabNet/Municipal Health Department of the City of São Paulo [22].*

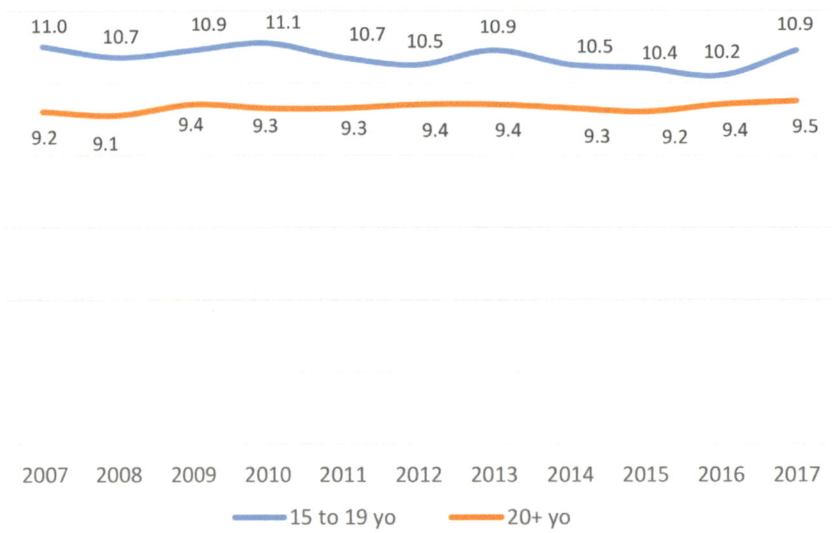


**Figure 3.**
*Low birth weight (<2.500 kg) for mothers between 15 and 19 years, and mothers older than 20 years, in the city of São Paulo between 2007 and 2017. Source: DATASUS/TabNet/Municipal Health Department of the City of São Paulo/Accessed July 15, 2018. Organized by: Centre for the Study of Violence of University of São Paulo.*

of pregnancies in the city of São Paulo between 2007 and 2017 lasted between 37 and 41 weeks—that is, they went to term for both the population of 15–19-year olds (87.7%) and for the population older than 20 (89.0%). Comparing these two groups also showed no major difference in relation to premature births (where gestation lasts less than 36 weeks). General data for the city show that, during the 2007–2017 period, babies born at less than 36 weeks accounted on average for 10.9% of births to mothers between 15 and 19 years, and 10% for mothers older than 20 [22].

With regard to the number of children with low birth weight, there is a slight variation between adolescent mothers and mothers older than 20. During the 2007–2017 period, in the city of São Paulo, the proportion of children with low birth weight (less than 2.500 kg) was 10.7% among 15–19-year-old mothers, and 9.3% for children born to mothers older than 20 (**Figure 3**).

Therefore, denaturalizing the view that adolescent pregnancy is a problem is essential to changing the discourse and, above all, rethinking practices related to pregnancy and motherhood during this period of life. This is not to say that the phenomenon should be treated as something normal, because it is not—but neither is it something abnormal. The proposition here is that we should discuss this matter outside of the scope of a universalizing and naturalizing view of normal/abnormal in order to seek out a new way of thinking that will allow for more humanized practices [15].

## 4. The Health Infancy project

The data that will be discussed below are from the Health Infancy project, an initiative by the Nucleus for the Study of Violence at the University of São Paulo (NEV-USP) that seeks to promote the healthy development of children born to teen mothers (13–19 years) starting at gestation all the way to 2 years of age. Through weekly home visits, participants received guidance about various issues related to gestation and infant development and were able to discuss with the visitors any questions or problems they had related to maternity. The strength of the project lies precisely in the relationship that is established between the adolescent and the visitor—who is also a mother from the same community—trained not only to transmit information but primarily to pay attention to the demands of the participant and her child in order to hear them out and address their anxieties and fears during this phase [23].

We opted to organize the discussion into topics and, based on both statistical data and concrete examples shared by the adolescents, reflect on how the proposals included in the health policies are carried out in day-to-day activities. We know that public policies will never fully account for the diversity of real-life situations; nevertheless, it is necessary to permanently improve policies in order to ensure their effectiveness as much as possible.

The Health Infancy project has been carried out since 2009 in the Jardim Ângela neighborhood in the southeast region of the city of São Paulo. In the 1990s, this region was considered by the United Nations to be the most violent urban region in the world, and currently still ranks among the city's most vulnerable neighborhoods. Nevertheless, the region has access to a free public health system and, at least in terms of prenatal, delivery, and infant care, the population is served by 18 UBSs, 2 emergency rooms, and 1 hospital.

In comparison with other regions of the city of São Paulo, Jardim Ângela is the sixth largest in terms of the number of pregnant adolescents. Rates are not only higher than the average for the city, but also present the greatest variation. Between 2003 and 2017, the rate of pregnant adolescents between 15 and 19 years of age in Jardim Ângela averaged 6.8%. In the graph below, we can see that during this period the rate was stable between 2003 and 2008, rose between 2009 and 2014, and fell starting in 2015 (**Figure 4**).

### 4.1 Finding out about pregnancy and utilizing health services

When a woman finds out she is pregnant, this represents a formative moment in any woman's life. When this woman is an adolescent, right away the perception is that the pregnancy was unplanned and as a result it will be badly received, especially by the girl's family. However, despite the initial shock upon receiving the news, and concern about how life will be from that moment onward, it was common for adolescents to say that they desired to be mothers, and for them to demonstrate happiness and satisfaction with the pregnancy. Furthermore, even in those

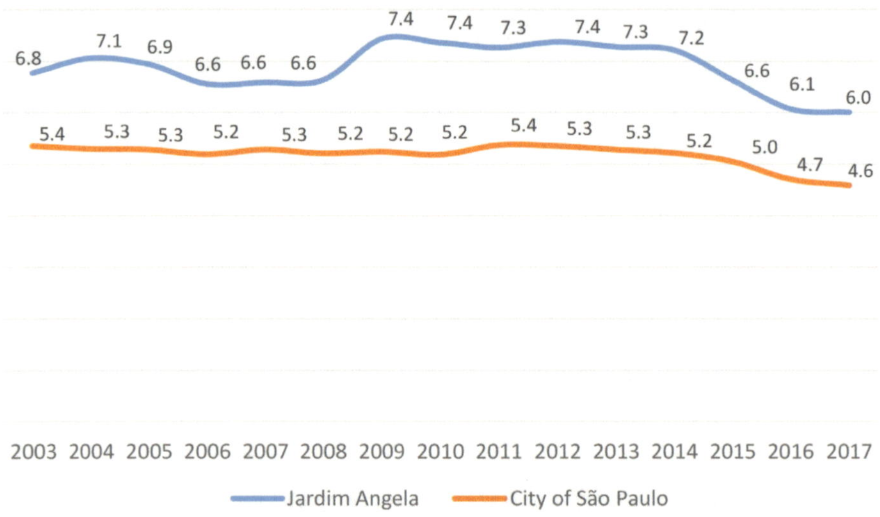


**Figure 4.**
*Comparison between average rates of pregnant adolescents in Jardim Ângela and in São Paulo. Source: DATASUS/TabNet/Municipal Health Department of the City of São Paulo/Accessed July 16, 2018. Organized by: Centre for the Study of Violence of University of São Paulo.*

cases where the family expressed dismay with the news of the pregnancy, primarily because they knew the difficulties that would be faced—lack of economic resources, dropping out of school and the subsequent problems in entering the labor market, and the adolescent's lack of maturity to care for a baby, among others—soon there was acceptance and increasing family support. It is also worth noting that in many cases, the adolescent had already left her parents' home and lived with her partner and the child's father, such was the couple's desire to have children [15, 24].

Still, the common perception that adolescent pregnancy is always unwanted and unplanned is oftentimes also held by health professionals. The discourse is usually focused on the negative repercussions of the pregnancy, both for the mother and for the child, and also for society as a whole. Knowledge and practices linked to adolescent pregnancy tend to be activated from the perception of risk. Therefore, upon reaching the UBS to confirm that they are pregnant, many adolescents say that they suffer negative or prejudiced comments. This reaction by health professionals runs counter to the stance proposed by humanized services, in that they do not welcome reproductive demands or recognize the adolescent as a holder of rights capable of making autonomous decisions [15].

Starting in 2012, the city of São Paulo's Department of Health began to publish data about the month of pregnancy during which prenatal consultations began. The large majority of pregnant women began to have consultations during the first 3 months of pregnancy. However, some differences were noted between women aged 15–19 and women older than 20. During the 2012–2017 period, we noted that pregnant women older than 20 began to visit the doctor earlier than pregnant women between 15 and 19. Among pregnant women older than 20, 84.1% began prenatal care during the first 3 months: 30.3% starting in the first month, 36.8% during the second month, and 17% during the third month. Among pregnant women aged 15–19, 73.6% began prenatal care during the first 3 months: 17.8% during the first month of pregnancy, 34.2% during the second month, and 21.6% during the third month [22].

Similar to what happened in the city as a whole, the Jardim Ângela neighborhood saw the large majority of pregnant women begin their prenatal consultations during the first trimester. Among pregnant women older than 20, 86.4% had prenatal

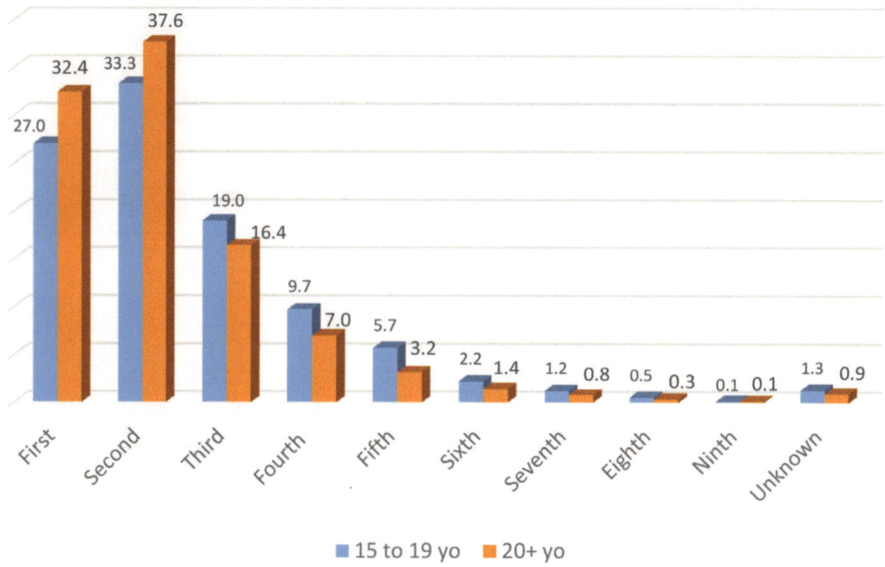


**Figure 5.**
*Percentage of pregnant women who carried out prenatal consultation in Jardim Ângela, by month. Source: DATASUS/TabNet/Municipal Health Department of the City of São Paulo/Accessed Jul 16, 2018. Organized by: Centre for the Study of Violence of University of São Paulo.*

consultations during the first trimester: 32.4% during the first month, 37.6% during the second month, and 16.4% during the third. Among pregnant women aged 15–19, 79.3% began prenatal consultations during the first trimester: 27% during the first month, 33.3% during the second, and 19% during the third month (**Figure 5**).

Comparing these data to citywide data, we note that the figures for both groups are higher than the city average. We also note that, similar to what happens in the city as a whole, in Jardim Ângela, pregnant women older than 20 tend to start their prenatal visits earlier than pregnant women aged 15–19. On the other hand, in Jardim Ângela, there is a larger proportion of pregnant women aged 15–19 who start receiving prenatal care during the first month of pregnancy.

### 4.2 Prenatal

We know that proper accompaniment during the prenatal period and delivery is fundamental for ensuring adequate conditions of survival for mothers and their babies [25]. The São Paulo Municipal Secretariat of Health, in accordance with federal policies, establishes that pregnant women should have monthly consultations (or at least 7), lab and ultrasound exams, free transportation vouchers to and from the exams and consultations, and visits before delivery. Furthermore, prenatal care should include spaces where mothers can voice their questions, worries, and difficulties; receive emotional support and encouragement to breastfeed, including time to exchange tips with other mothers; and also include the involvement of family members and community members in this process [12].

In the city of São Paulo, pregnant women who have seven or more prenatal visits not only represent the majority, but their numbers have been climbing over the years. However, when comparing data for the group of 15–19-year olds to those older than 20, we note some differences. In the 2007–2017 period, 77.6% of women older than 20 had seven or more prenatal visits, while 64% of those between 15 and 19 did so. For pregnant women older than 20, 17.1% had 4–6 prenatal consultations, compared with 26.5% for women aged 15–19 (**Figure 6**).

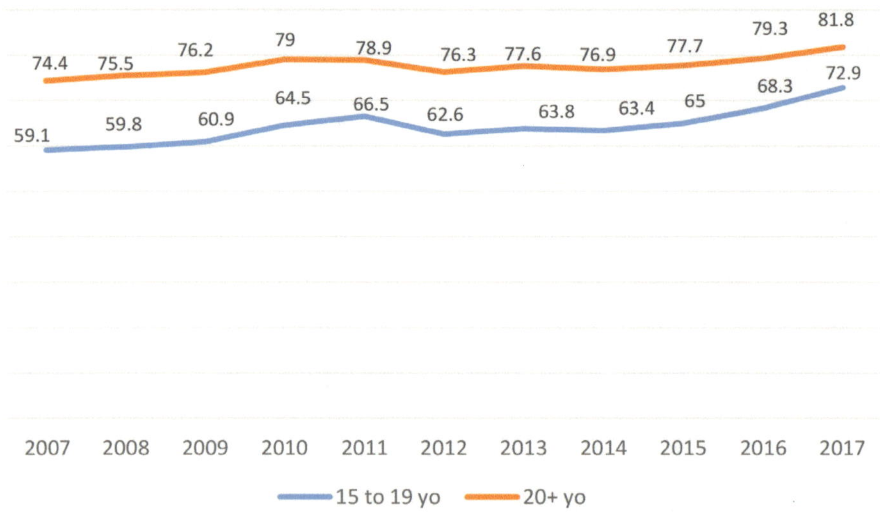


**Figure 6.**
*Percentage of pregnant women who had seven or more prenatal consultations, for 15–19-year olds and for women older than 20 in the city of São Paulo. Source: DATASUS/TabNet/Municipal Health Department of the City of São Paulo/Accessed Jul 16, 2018. Organized by: Centre for the Study of Violence of University of São Paulo.*

When we look at data from Jardim Ângela and compare them with those for the city, we note that pregnant women who had seven or more prenatal visits also are the majority, and that Jardim Ângela women report higher rates than the average for the city over the same period. We also see the same difference between women aged 15–19 and women older than 20. Pregnant women older than 20 more frequently had seven or more consultations (81.4%) than those aged 15–19 (74.3%). Women who had 4–6 visits accounted for 14.8% of pregnant women older than 20, and 19.9% of those aged 15–19 (**Figure** 7).

Among the adolescents accompanied by the Health Infancy project, more than 90% had prenatal exams at the UBS closest to their home. In general, there were no reports of difficulty in accessing this kind of service, nor in carrying out the exams—except ultrasounds, which have a long wait time. In this sense, then, there seems to be a compatibility between what is proposed and what is in fact accessed by the population. What still needs to be debated is the quality of these services. The adolescents say that they were well received, especially by the nurses, but they also complained about this relationship oftentimes being merely prescriptive, that the health professionals' recommendations were not fully understood, that the pregnant women were not welcomed, and in some cases they noted a prejudiced tone in the health professionals' attitudes [15].

The fact that they are adolescents reinforces the hierarchy of those who know—the professional—and those who need knowledge—the adolescent—which creates difficulties for the building of a more horizontal relationship. Oftentimes, out of fear or embarrassment, the adolescents failed to ask questions or to follow the recommended guidelines, which could impact the baby's development. In this sense, it is of utmost importance that the health professionals be aware of the peculiarities of this kind of assistance [26].

### 4.3 Childbirth

The moment of childbirth is the one most feared by adolescents. Although prenatal consultations provide a space for them to prepare themselves for delivery,

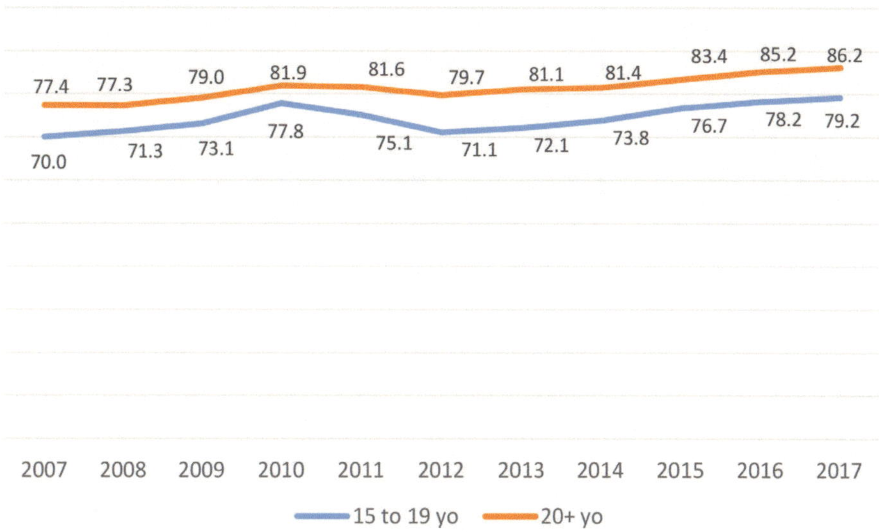


**Figure 7.**
*Percentage of pregnant women who had seven or more prenatal consultations, for women aged 15–19, and for women older than 20 in Jardim Ângela. Source: DATASUS/TabNet/Municipal Health Department of the City of São Paulo/Accessed Jul 16, 2018. Organized by: Centre for the Study of Violence of University of São Paulo.*

what we see in practice is that the matter is little discussed, as are the fears and anxieties that surround this moment. In general, adolescents know that two forms of childbirth are possible—vaginal and caesarian section—and about the benefits of vaginal delivery; but the fear of the pain, the initial signs of labor, the procedures carried out—these are not discussed very much [15, 26].

It was clear from the accounts given by adolescents to the visitors that certain comments and attitudes of some health professionals contributed even more to the suffering they underwent during delivery. Not rarely, the sensations that the adolescents felt upon being admitted to the hospital were dismissed by the hospital staff, there were accounts of verbal humiliation, and the adolescents' knowledge about their own bodies were disregarded, especially in relation to labor pains [15].

Another aspect that merits attention is that of going from hospital to hospital during labor, which could lead to serious risks for the mother and the baby. Many adolescents reported having to change hospital due to a lack of beds; and so, in addition to not being able to deliver the baby in the hospital they had planned for—as the law stipulates— and in addition to suffering from uncertainty about the unknown, there were also risks of possible consequences to their health.

One aspect that came to our attention is the difference in the delivery experience for pregnant women aged 15–19 and for those older than 20. Although the country is undergoing an epidemic of scheduled caesarian sections—which creates risks for the mother and the baby—we note that, in the city of São Paulo, between 2007 and 2017 the most common form of childbirth for women between 15 and 19 was vaginal (73.3%) [22].

We also noted that during the course of this period, these trends remained steady for both groups. Among pregnant women older than 20, the proportion of cesarean sections not only remained higher than 50% during the course of this period, but it also rose between 2007 and 2013, after which it again declined (**Figure 8**). Among pregnant women aged 15–19, vaginal birth remained close to 70% during this entire period, and in 2015 began to climb, reaching 73.3% of births in 2017 (**Figure 9**).

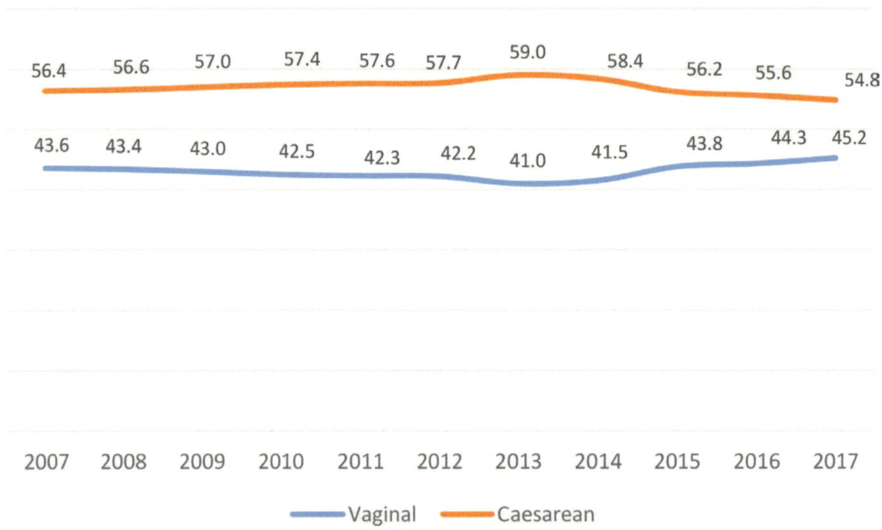


**Figure 8.**
*Cesarian births × vaginal births for pregnant women older than 20, between 2007 and 2017 in the city of São Paulo. Source: DATASUS/TabNet/Municipal Health Department of the City of São Paulo/Accessed Jul 16, 2018. Organized by: Centre for the Study of Violence of University of São Paulo.*

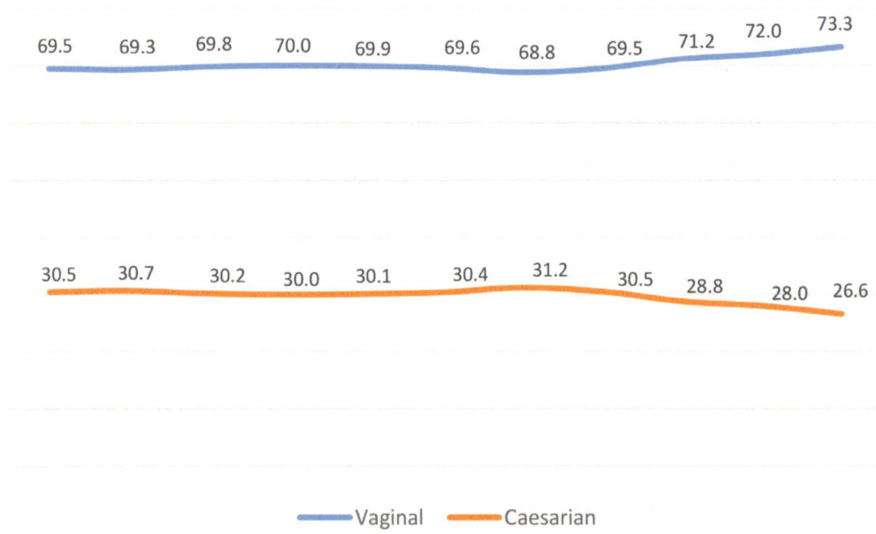


**Figure 9.**
*Cesarian births × vaginal births for pregnant women aged 15–19 years, between 2007 and 2017 in the city of São Paulo. Source: DATASUS/TabNet/Municipal Health Department of the City of São Paulo/Accessed Jul 16, 2018. Organized by: Centre for the Study of Violence of University of São Paulo.*

Unlike what happens in the city as a whole, vaginal births were the most common form of birth in Jardim Ângela, for both age groups. In 2017, the rate of vaginal births was 55.6% for women older than 20, and 76.1% for women aged 15–19 years. This difference reinforces what studies have already shown about the difference in public and private services in terms of choosing the delivery method, in that at some private hospitals the rate of C-sections surpasses 90%. Because we are dealing with a poor peripheral district of the city, with little access to private services, the rate of vaginal births is higher than for the rest of the city.

### 4.4 Accompaniment of child development

While there were few difficulties in receiving prenatal care, the same cannot be said for accompaniment of the baby. It was very common for adolescents in the project to mention that they had difficulties scheduling the child's routine visits to the doctor, and a lack of pediatricians present at health posts [15].

During the course of the visits it was also very common for the adolescents to complain about not receiving guidance about the development of their children, with no knowledge about forms of stimulating their development and many questions about whether their child's development was normal for their age—at how many months should the child start crawling, walking, talking, etc. The consultations were focused strictly on anthropometric measures and more serious health problems, with no focus on promoting holistic development, which would include an eye for the development of motor, cognitive, and socio-affective skills [15, 27].

In this sense, one of the main focuses of the Health Infancy project was precisely on discussing with the adolescents what they should expect during each phase of their child's development, and what kind of activities could stimulate their child, while also stressing that each child has their own pace of development [23].

Another aspect that led to many questions was in regard to children's feeding habits, an essential aspect for healthy childhood development but one which was little discussed in routine visits. Theoretically, this subject should be discussed as soon as prenatal care begins, because the mother's eating habits will directly affect the way that she will feed her child.

## 5. Conclusions

We note that in recent decades, governments—together with society—have been making a concerted effort to improve services to mothers and children. Between the period of 1990 and 2015, Brazil reduced the maternal mortality rate by 56%, to 62 deaths per 100,000 births, from 143. And the infant mortality rate dropped to 13 per 1000 live births, from 62 during the same period [22].

Despite progress, the levels of mortality are still high when compared with other countries that have similar levels of economic development. Therefore, it is increasingly critical that Brazil's public policies include integrated actions, and not isolated and verticalized measures, in order to effectively promote maternal-infant health.

Universality, equity, and integrality are the guiding directives of the SUS. However, access to health services and activities are not always guaranteed to everyone, and it is even more difficult to access services that meet the specific needs of the population and take into account all dimensions of the individual.

In this sense, it is necessary to continue investing in the creation of health policies and services capable of meeting real needs, capable of encouraging social opportunity, and capable of reinforcing women's autonomy and the rights of children and adolescents.

## Author details

Aline Mizutani Gomes and Renato Alves*
Center for the Study of Violence, University of São Paulo, Brazil

*Address all correspondence to: ralves@usp.br

## References

[1] Instituto Brasileiro de Geografia e Estatística. Séries estatísticas & séries históricas. Rio de Janeiro: O Instituto. 2018. Available from: http://www.ibge.gov.br/series_estatisticas/ [Accessed: 10 July 2018]

[2] Paim J, Travassos C, Almeida C, Bahia L, Macinko J. O sistema de saúde brasileiro: história, avanços e desafios. Lancet. 2011;**377**:1778-1797. DOI: 10.1016/S0140-6736(11)60054-8

[3] Menicucci T. História da reforma sanitária brasileira e do Sistema Único de Saúde: mudanças, continuidades e a agenda atual. História, Ciências, Saúde. 2014;**21**:77-92. DOI: 10.1590/S0104-59702014000100004

[4] Visão Mundial. Estudo sobre as políticas públicas de proteção à saúde infantil e materna no brasil: um olhar especial para os filhos de mães adolescentes. Recife: Visão Mundial. 2011

[5] Brasil. Presidência da República. Lei nº 8.069, de 13 de julho de 1990. Dispõe sobre o Estatuto da Criança e do Adolescente e dá outras providências. Brasília: Diário Oficial da União 16 jul 1990. Available from: http://www.planalto.gov.br/ccivil_03/LEIS/L8069.htm. [Accessed: 12 July 2018]

[6] Brasil. Ministério do Desenvolvimento Social e Combate à Fome. Secretaria Nacional de Renda de Cidadania. Bolsa Família: transferência de renda e apoio à família no acesso à saúde, à educação e à assistência social. Brasília: Ministério do Desenvolvimento Social e Combate à Fome. Secretaria Nacional de Renda de Cidadania, 2015.

[7] Brasil. Ministério da Saúde. Portaria nº 2.488/GM/MS, de 24 de outubro de 2011. Aprova a Política Nacional de Atenção Básica, estabelecendo a revisão de diretrizes e normas para a organização da Atenção Básica, para a Estratégia Saúde da Família (ESF) e o Programa de Agentes Comunitários de Saúde (PACS). Brasília: Diário Oficial da União 22 out 2011. Available from: http://bvsms.saude.gov.br/bvs/saudelegis/gm/2011/prt2488_21_10_2011.html. [Accessed: 15 July 2018]

[8] Brasil. Ministério da Saúde. Secretaria de Atenção à Saúde. Departamento de Atenção Básica. Política Nacional de Atenção Básica/Ministério da Saúde. Secretaria de Atenção à Saúde. Departamento de Atenção Básica. Brasília: Ministério da Saúde; 2012

[9] Brasil. Ministério da Saúde. Secretaria de Atenção à Saúde. Departamento de Ações Programáticas Estratégicas. *Política nacional de atenção integral à saúde da mulher*: princípios e diretrizes. Brasília: DF; 2004

[10] Serruya SJ, Cecatti JG, Lago TDG. O programa de Humanização do Parto e Nascimento do Ministério da Saúde. Caderno de Saúde Pública. 2004;**5**(20):1281-1289

[11] Fortes PAC. Ética, direitos dos usuários e políticas de humanização da atenção à saúde. Saúde e Sociedade [online]. 2004;**13**(3):30-35. DOI: 10.1590/S0104-12902004000300004

[12] Brasil, Ministério da Saúde. PORTARIA Nº 1.459, DE 24 DE JUNHO DE 2011. Institui, no âmbito do Sistema Único de Saúde - SUS - a Rede Cegonha. Brasília: Diário Oficial da União 25 jun 2011. Available from: http://bvsms.saude.gov.br/bvs/saudelegis/gm/2011/prt1459_24_06_2011.html. [Accessed: 15 July 2018]

[13] Martin JA, Hamilton BE, Osterman MJK, et al. Births: Final Data for 2015. National Vital Statistics Report; Vol. 66, No 1. Hyattsville, MD: National Center

for Health Statistics; 2017. Available from: https://www.unicef.org/panama/spanish/EmbarazoAdolescente_ESP(1).pdf [Accessed: 07 October 2018]

[14] Organización Panamericana de la Salud. Acelerar el progreso hacia la reducción del embarazo en la adolescencia en América Latina y el Caribe. Washington, DC: Fondo de Población de las Naciones Unidas y Fondo de las Naciones Unidas para la Infancia; 2018

[15] Alves RA. O Processo de Desenvolvimento de um Programa de Visitação Domiciliar para Adolescentes Gestantes e Mães. São Paulo: Instituto de Psicologia da Universidade de São Paulo; 2014

[16] Pantoja ALN. Ser alguém na vida: uma análise sócio-antropológica da gravidez/maternidade na adolescência, em Belém do Pará, Brasil. Cadernos de Saúde Pública. 2003;**19**(suppl. 2): S335-S343

[17] Katz RA. Adolescentes e maternidade: um destino, um problema, uma escolha? Rio de Janeiro: Instituto Fernandes Figueira, Fundação Oswaldo Cruz; 1999

[18] Heilborn ML, Salem T, Rohden F, Brandão E, Knauth D, Víctora C, et al. Aproximações socioantropológicas sobre gravidez na adolescência. Horizontes Antropológicos. 2002;**8**(17):13-45

[19] Barbosa AM. Análise sociodemográfica da fecundidade de adolescentes e jovens no Brasil: 1970/2006. Trabalho apresentado no XVI Encontro Nacional de Estudos Populacionais, realizado em Caxambu-MG—Brasil, de 29 de setembro a 03 de outubro de 2008

[20] Coll A. Embarazo en la adolescencia? Cuál es el problema? In: Burak SD. Adolescencia y juventud en América Latina; Costa Rica: LUR; 2001. pp. 425-445

[21] Gomes R, Fonseca EMGO, Veiga AJMO. A visão da pediatria acerca da gravidez na adolescência: um estudo bibliográfico. Revista Latino-Americana de Enfermagem. 2002;**10**(3):408-414

[22] Municipal Health Department of the City of São Paulo. DATASUS. TabNet. 2018. Organized by: Centre for the Study of Violence of University of São Paulo. [Accessed: 14 July 2018]

[23] Cardia N, Alves R, Gomes AM, Mourão A. Home visitation programs for early child development: Experiences in Latin America and the Caribbean. In: Roggman LA, Cardia N, editors. Home Visitation Programs. Basel, Switzerland: Springer International Publishing; 2016. pp. 157-189. DOI: 10.1007/978-3-319-17984-1

[24] Estrada F, Suárez-López L, Hubert C, Allen-Leigh B, Campero L, Cruz-Jimenez L. Factors associated with desire pregnancy among adolescent women in five Latin American countries: a multilevel analysis. BJOG. 2018;**125**(10):1330-1336. DOI: 10.1111/1471-0528.15313

[25] Celhay P, Johannsen J, Martinez S, Vidal C. Paying patients for prenatal care: The effect of a small cash transfer on stillbirths and survival, IDB Working Paper Series, No. IDB-WP-817. Washington, DC: Inter-American Development Bank (IDB); 2017

[26] Luz NF, Assis TR, Rezende FR. Puérperas adolescentes: percepções relacionadas ao pré-natal e ao parto. Goiás: ABCS Health Sciences. 2015;**40**(2):80-84

[27] Black MM, Walker SP, Fernald LC, et al. Early childhood development coming of age: Science through the life course. The Lancet. 2016;**389**(10064):77-90. DOI: 10.1016/S0140-6736(16)31389-7

Chapter 3

# Cytokines and Maternal Omega-3 LCPUFAs Supplementation

*Yessica Rodriguez-Santana and Luis Peña-Quintana*

## Abstract

Daily supplementation of maternal diet during pregnancy and lactation with a fish oil-enriched dairy product increases the percentage of DHA and other omega-3 (ω-3) long-chain polyunsaturated fatty acids (LCPUFAs) in mothers (placenta, plasma, erythrocyte membranes, and breast milk) and children (plasma and erythrocyte membranes). This supplementation during critical periods such as pregnancy, lactation, and early development of a newborn may influence the levels of certain inflammatory cytokines, reducing pro-inflammatory cytokines and promoting an anti-inflammatory "environment". In pregnant women who have not received any supplement of omega-3 LCPUFAs, IL-6 plasma levels are higher, while TNF-alpha plasma levels are also higher in their breastfed infant at birth and 2 months thereafter. There could be a relationship between docosahexaenoic acid (DHA) and the concentrations of different cytokines.

**Keywords:** docosahexaenoic acid (DHA), eicosapentaenoic acid (EPA), omega-3 LCPUFAs, pregnancy, lactation, cytokines, fatty acids

## 1. Introduction

Interest in the therapeutic effects of omega-3 (ω-3) fatty acids has grown over the last 30 years, particularly in regard to visual and neurological development in newborns, the immune system, and inflammatory and cardiovascular diseases [1–9].

Inflammation is one of the principal causes of complications during pregnancy and of prematurity and neonatal morbidity [10–15].

Docosahexaenoic acid (DHA) has anti-inflammatory effects and can alter the production of inflammatory cytokines in animal models, cell culture, and in humans [16–26]. A high intake of omega-3 fatty acids has been associated with a reduction in arachidonic acid-derived inflammatory eicosanoids, cytokine production, reactive oxygen species, and expression of adhesion molecules [27]. It is also associated with the production of lipid mediators [28] that have anti-inflammatory [29–31] and immunomodulatory effects [27]. Both eicosapentaenoic acid (EPA) and DHA affect the function of many immune cells and can have a beneficial effect in preventing inflammatory or immune-mediated diseases, but their effects and mechanisms of action can differ [32]. They can inhibit the production of pro-inflammatory cytokines such as tumour necrosis factor-alpha and interleukin (IL)-1 and IL-6 [33]. In animal models their intake during pregnancy appears to exert an anti-inflammatory effect on damaged tissue in the young [34–36], while in humans it produces a decrease in Th1 cytokines such as interferon-gamma (IFN-γ) and IL-1 in infants' plasma and a decrease in the Th2 cytokines IL-14 and IL-13 in the umbilical cord blood [32, 37].

## 2. Omega-3 fatty acids

Long-chain polyunsaturated fatty acids are fatty acids containing at least 18–20 carbon atoms. They are categorised into two main families according to the position of the first double bond [38], as either omega-3 series or omega-6 series. In omega-3 fatty acids, the first double bond is between the third and fourth carbon atoms (**Table 1**).

The most relevant omega-3 LCPUFAs are alpha-linolenic acid (ALA), docosahexaenoic acid, eicosapentaenoic acid, and docosapentaenoic acid (DPA), while the most relevant omega-6 LCPUFAs are linoleic acid (LA) and arachidonic acid (ARA).

### 2.1 Synthesis and sources of fatty acids

In humans, the synthesis of omega-3 and omega-6 fatty acids is limited; they are therefore considered essential fatty acids. LA and ALA are synthesised in large quantities in plants, but humans and other mammals cannot make them from their precursor, oleic acid, because they lack the active enzymes Δ-12 and Δ-15 desaturase [38]. Humans can synthesise other long-chain fatty acids such as ARA, DHA, and EPA from LA and ALA, which are precursors to the omega-6 and omega-3 series, respectively. However, conversion of these fatty acids to DHA, EPA, and ARA is inefficient [39], the most efficient method being to obtain them from the diet. Conversion can vary between sexes and is more efficient in women [40]. It increases during pregnancy and is reduced in newborns [40] due to their lower enzymatic activity.

Both omega-3 and omega-6 LCPUFA syntheses occur via the same pathway of elongation, desaturation, and peroxisomal retroconversion [41]. The most important enzymes in the desaturation processes are Δ-5 and Δ-6 desaturase. The two precursors, LA and ALA, compete for Δ-6 desaturase, but the enzyme has a greater affinity for ALA [40]. Therefore, a high supply of ALA causes a reduction in the synthesis of LA derivatives. In contrast, if LA supply is greater than ALA supply, conversion of ALA to its derivatives is limited. The Western diet contains 10–20 times more omega-6 than omega-3 fatty acids [41]. In addition, the fatty acid content of plasma and many other tissues comprises predominantly omega-6 fatty acids, with the exception of the brain and retina, which are rich in omega-3 [41]. Thus, a high intake of EPA and DHA results in a decrease in tissue levels of ARA and an increase in EPA and DHA, due to enzymatic competition between the two series [42].

| | |
|---|---|
| Omega-6 fatty acids | Linoleic acid (LA) C18:2 ω-6 |
| | Arachidonic acid (ARA) C20:4ω-6 |
| Omega-3 fatty acids | Alpha linolenic acid (ALA) C18:3 ω-3 |
| | Eicosapentaenoic acid (EPA) C20:5 ω-3 |
| | Docosahexaenoic acid (DHA) C22:6 ω-3 |
| | Docosapentaenoic acid (DPA) C22:5 ω-3 |

**Table 1.**
*Omega-6 and omega-3 long-chain polyunsaturated fatty acids.*

Polyunsaturated fatty acids are found mainly in oily fish and in seed oils. LA, the precursor of omega-6 fatty acids, is present in soybean, corn, and sunflower oils, while ALA, the precursor to omega-3 fatty acids, is found in numerous vegetables, such as linseed, canola, pumpkin seeds, and walnuts. The main dietary sources of EPA and DHA are cold-water oily fish (e.g. sardines, salmon, mackerel, and herring) [43] (**Figure 1**).

Despite the benefits of a diet rich in omega-3 fatty acids, there is no consensus on their recommended daily intake. The dietary recommendations from national and international bodies on the intake of omega-3 long-chain fatty acids, in particular EPA and DHA, vary between 200 and 600 mg per day for adults and 40 and 250 mg per day for infants older than 6 months, children, and adolescents [42]. These recommendations are based on the observed association between the omega-3 fatty acid consumption and reduced risk of cardiovascular disease. According to the Nutrition Committee of American Heart Association (AHA Nutrition Committee) recommendations, eating at least two servings of fish per week or 500 mg per day of omega-3 LCPUFAs prevents and reduces the risk of cardiac disease [44, 45]. The expert panel of the European Food Safety Authority (EFSA) recommends an intake of 250 mg per day of omega-3 LCPUFAs, in contrast to the Australian suggested dietary targets of 610 mg EPA and 430 mg DHA per day in adults to reduce cardiovascular risk [38, 46, 47]. To achieve an anti-inflammatory effect, it is recommended to eat between 500 and 1000 mg of omega-3 fatty acids per day [48]. There are also specific recommendations for certain population groups: in pregnant or breastfeeding women, an additional intake of 100–200 mg DHA per day is recommended to compensate for oxidative losses of DHA and its accumulation in the foetus [42].

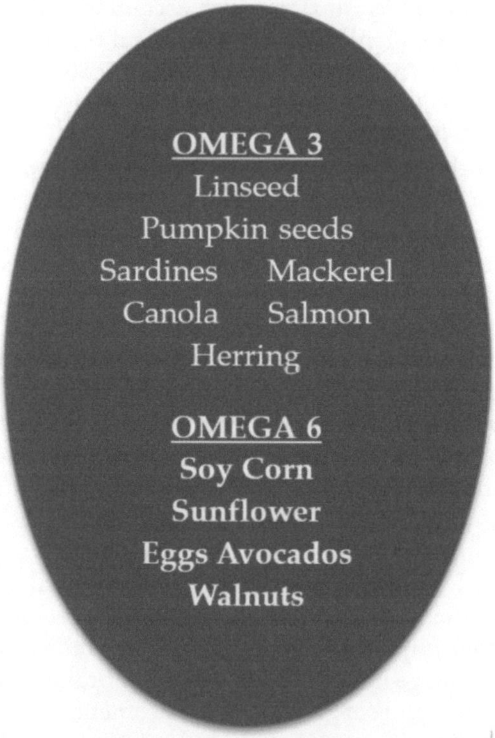
OMEGA 3
Linseed
Pumpkin seeds
Sardines Mackerel
Canola Salmon
Herring
OMEGA 6
Soy Corn
Sunflower
Eggs Avocados
Walnuts

**Figure 1.**
*LCPUFAs food sources.*

There are few data on the adverse effects of long-term high-dose DHA supplementation. The EFSA expert panel considers DHA dietary supplementation of up to 1 g per day to not pose a risk in the general population. In a systematic review [1] of studies on DHA supplements during pregnancy, it was concluded that an intake of 1–2.7 g per day of omega-3 LCPUFAs is not harmful.

## 2.2 General functions of fatty acids

### *2.2.1 Cell membrane structure and function*

Omega-3 polyunsaturated fatty acids are important structural components of cell membranes, where they are present as membrane phospholipids (esterified fatty acids) or as free molecules [49]. The incorporation of free polyunsaturated fatty acids into membrane phospholipids appears to alter the physical properties of the membranes. They can influence the structure of membrane phospholipids, reducing the van der Waals interactions [50].

They contribute to several membrane functions such as fluidity, permeability, enzymatic and receptor activity, gene expression, and signal transduction [41, 42, 51]. The changes in permeability appear to depend directly on the degree of fatty acid desaturation [49]. EPA and DHA are of particular biological importance.

### *2.2.2 Visual and neurological function*

The nervous system takes a long time to develop and mature, but there are many crucial events that occur during pregnancy and the first years of life. The brain grows rapidly between week 20 of gestation and 2 years of age, increasing in size by 64% during the first 3 months of life [52]. In these stages there is a period termed the *window of sensitivity*, during which certain nutrients or stimuli can influence and promote neurological development and functional brain capacity. Several nutrients have been described to play a crucial role in the development of the nervous system, including choline, iron, zinc, and long-chain fatty acids such as nervonic acid and DHA [53–55].

DHA forms part of the structural lipids of cell membranes, particularly the phospholipids found in the nervous tissue and the retina [38], where high levels of DHA have been found, primarily in the grey matter and photoreceptors; it is therefore thought to be essential for proper neurological and visual development [9, 35, 56–58]. Similarly, high levels of omega-3 polyunsaturated fatty acids have been found in the basal ganglia, frontal cortex, occipital cortex, hippocampus, and thalamus in studies performed on the young of baboons and rats, which suggests that they affect sensory-motor integration and memory [59–61]. Cerebral development affects cognitive, social, and motor functions and communication. Stimulation and optimal nutrition [62] are essential. It has been demonstrated that babies who receive adequate quantities of omega-3 LCPUFAs, especially of DHA, show better development in these areas [63–68], so DHA is thought to be essential for the growth and function of neuronal and visual tissue [53]. These benefits continue beyond childhood [64, 69], and DHA is recommended as an essential dietary component in breastfeeding women and in children, to support brain development [54].

DHA appears to have important properties as a free radical scavenger, protecting against oxidative damage in developing and adult brains. It also has a role in neuronal plasticity, a process that allows the replacement of damaged neuronal circuits and reorganisation of existing ones. It combines with glycerophosphocholine and phosphatidylserine to promote the formation of membrane phospholipids for the growth of nerve cells [55] and has also been observed to play a role in cell migration during brain development [70]. Animal studies have demonstrated that DHA supplementation during pregnancy and breastfeeding is associated with an increased density of dendritic spines in the hippocampus [71] and of some synaptic proteins in the brains of weaned rats, while DHA deficiency has been associated with smaller neuronal soma [72] and altered synaptic vesicle density and neuronal growth and survival. Another study has demonstrated that supplementation with DHA significantly increases neuronal growth and synaptogenesis and increases levels of pre- and postsynaptic proteins involved in synaptic transmission and long-term potentiation, which is associated with improved synaptic function [73].

### 2.2.3 DHA and oxidative stress

Omega-3 fatty acids are considered effective in the prevention of many diseases due to their antioxidant effects [74], yet there remains some debate on the subject. DHA, being a highly unsaturated fatty acid, is extremely susceptible to lipid peroxidation. Therefore, it is essential to ensure that LCPUFA supplements are safe, as they may generate free radicals that can affect the tissues. However, several studies in children found no abnormalities in baseline levels of peroxidised lipids nor in antioxidant enzymatic activity. Randomised studies in which up to 1 g per day of DHA or 2–7 g per day of omega-3 LCPUFAs was given found no adverse effects, including in pregnant women [75, 76].

Pregnancy is a state in which there is a high metabolic demand and increased production of free radicals. Pregnant women have been observed to have higher levels of free radical damage than non-pregnant women. Labour also involves increased oxidative damage in both mother and baby, being even higher in premature newborns [77, 78]. Studies carried out in animals have found increased activity of superoxide dismutase (SOD), an important antioxidant enzyme, in rat brains following post-natal DHA supplementation [79]. In a subsequent study in pregnant women, it was suggested that consumption of fish oil during pregnancy could have antioxidant effects during this period although the results were not conclusive [80].

### 2.2.4 Other benefits and disease prevention

Several studies have demonstrated the beneficial effect of fatty acids in inflammatory [81, 82] and autoimmune diseases such as systemic lupus erythematosus [43], asthma, cystic fibrosis [83], chronic obstructive pulmonary disease (COPD) [38], rheumatoid arthritis [81], multiple sclerosis [33, 38, 84, 85], ulcerative colitis [86], Crohn's disease [81], and type 2 diabetes mellitus [33, 87].

The beneficial effects of omega-3 fatty acids on cardiovascular disease are widely known [88, 89]. Omega-3 LCPUFAs not only reduce triglyceride levels [90–93] but also reduce the production of chemotactic agents, growth factors, adhesion molecules, inflammatory eicosanoids and inflammatory cytokines, decrease blood pressure, increase nitric oxide production, improve endothelial relaxation and vascular compliance, and reduce thrombus formation and cardiac arrhythmias [94, 95]. Although the mechanisms of their protective effects are not fully established, it has been proposed that they may be due to the anti-inflammatory effects of these fatty acids on blood vessel walls [95], their aforementioned lipid-lowering effect, the regulated production of less potent eicosanoids, and the inhibition of pro-inflammatory cytokine production [89, 94], mechanisms which have also been shown to exert benefits in peripheral vascular disease [94].

Fish oil supplementation has also been shown to be beneficial in oncological processes [38] and is associated with a reduced incidence of metastatic breast cancer [33]. Its benefits have also been demonstrated in patients with colorectal cancer [96], with an observed reduction in inflammatory markers such as interleukin-6 (IL-6) in patients taking omega-3 fatty acid supplements, although these benefits are dependent on the duration, dose, and route of supplementation and the specific type of oncological treatment received. Its effects in leukaemia, lymphoma, neuroblastoma, glioblastoma, and lung, cervical, pancreatic, bladder, and ovarian cancer [97] have also been studied. The proposed mechanisms by which LCPUFAs act as adjuvants in cancer-specific treatments relate to their antitumour properties: they are anti-inflammatory [98], antiproliferative, pro-apoptotic, anti-invasive, and antimetastatic [99] and have epigenetic-regulatory effects [100]. Further studies are required to establish the therapeutic recommendations for EPA and DHA in oncological processes [97].

## 3. DHA and inflammation

Inflammation is part of the body's normal response to injury or infection. However, when it is uncontrolled or inappropriate, it can damage the body's own tissues, contributing to a wide variety of chronic and acute disorders. Inflammation is characterised by the production of inflammatory cytokines, ARA-derived eicosanoids (prostaglandins, thromboxanes, leukotrienes), reactive oxygen species (ROS), and molecular adhesion [81, 101].

The term *cytokine* encompasses a group of families of low molecular weight molecules that are structurally related and comprise more than 200 members. They are characterised by their ability to alter the functional activity of cells and tissues [102]. They are involved in the immunoregulatory and effector mechanisms of the innate and adaptive immune system. They are also involved in angiogenesis and have been found to play a key role in neuro-immune and neuroendocrine processes. Their pleiotropism makes their functional classification difficult, but they can be divided according to their most significant function into the following groups [103, 104]: adaptive immune mediators, innate immune mediators, haemopoiesis mediators, and pro-inflammatory and immunosuppressive cytokines.

In disease states, fish oil has been shown to act as an anti-inflammatory agent. Omega-3 fatty acids regulate the production of ARA-derived eicosanoids [81]. EPA competes with ARA to stimulate the production of series three prostaglandins and series five leukotrienes that have a lesser inflammatory action than ARA-derived eicosanoids. Supplementation with DHA leads to changes in the metabolism of ARA and in the balance of eicosanoids synthesised from omega-3 and omega-6 fatty acids. Thus it can affect the functions regulated by these eicosanoids [42].

Although fatty acids can modify the quantity and type of eicosanoids produced, they can also modify inflammation via eicosanoid-independent mechanisms that include acting on receptors, intracellular signalling pathways, and transcription factor activity [51]. They are able to reduce levels of C-reactive protein (CRP), cytokines [81], chemokines, and other inflammatory biomarkers. In addition, they produce the lipid mediators known as resolvins and protectins, which have anti-inflammatory and immunomodulatory effects [27–30, 43, 81]. Other anti-inflammatory actions of omega-3 LCPUFAs include a reduction in major histocompatibility complex (MHC) class II antigen presentation, reduction in reactive T cells, and reduction in Th1 cytokine production.

Omega-3 LCPUFAs could be said to act directly on inflammation by replacing arachidonic acid as a substrate for eicosanoid synthesis and indirectly by altering the expression of inflammatory genes via activation of transcription factors [101], among other mechanisms. The pathways are complex and much remains to be determined. It is thought that the nuclear factor (erythroid-derived 2)-like 2 (Nrf2) transcription factor plays a key role in the anti-inflammatory effects of DHA and EPA. Via Nrf2-dependent signalling, DHA can inhibit pro-inflammatory mediators such as nitric oxide synthase and cyclooxygenase-2 (COX-2) and pro-inflammatory cytokines such as IL-6, interleukin-1 (IL-1), and tumour necrosis factor-α (TNF-α) [33]. Other studies suggest that omega-3 LCPUFAs are natural ligands of peroxisome proliferator-activated receptor gamma (PPAR-γ), a transcription factor that regulates the expression of genes involved in cellular proliferation, inflammation, and metabolism of fatty acids and lipoproteins. Activation of PPAR-γ can inhibit nuclear factor kappa-light-chain-enhancer of activated B cells (NF-κB) signalling and expression of inflammatory genes [105]. Despite the available data, little is known about the cellular and molecular mechanisms by which omega-3 LCPUFAs exert their beneficial effect in the prevention of inflammatory and immune diseases [32]; such mechanisms are yet to be fully determined.

## 4. DHA in pregnancy and lactation

Essential fatty acids and those derived from LA (the omega-6 group) and ALA (the omega-3 group) play an important role during pregnancy. They have been associated with prolonged pregnancy, delay of spontaneous labour and reduction in recurrent premature labour in animal and human studies, improving neonatal outcomes [106]. In vulnerable states such as pregnancy and lactation, a high intake of omega-3 LCPUFAs is recommended as maternal levels of DHA decrease during pregnancy [1] and continue to decrease if the lactation period is long [107]. Maternal DHA levels have also been observed to decrease further in multiple pregnancies and are lower in multiparous than in primiparous women [108] and when the time between pregnancies is short. This could be explained by the high demand for these fatty acids during pregnancy as the foetus receives them preferentially via the placenta [109]. The foetus' DHA status depends exclusively on this transfer and in turn its supply in the mother's diet [110]. Indeed, omega-3 PUFA supplementation in pregnancy has been associated with increased DHA concentrations in the plasma, placenta, and umbilical cord blood [111].

Lactation is another period in which DHA consumption is beneficial for both the mother and child. Breast milk contains DHA, as well as omega-6 and other omega-3 LCPUFAs, which make up 2% of the total fatty acid content. It also contains components that play a specific immunological role such as cytokines, growth factors, leucocytes, immunoglobulins, lysosomes, and proteins such as lactoferrin. The presence of cytokines in breast milk helps the neonatal immune system develop and confers protection to the infant who does not yet have a network of mature cytokines [112]. Even at femtomolar concentrations, they can regulate the actions and properties of immune cells. A wide range of both pro-inflammatory and anti-inflammatory cytokines has been detected via numerous methods in breast milk throughout the different stages of lactation and includes IL-1 beta (β), IL-6, TNF-α, and transforming growth factor beta (TGF-β) [113].

The fatty acids present in breast milk also appear to play an important role in the maturation and function of the immune system. Exclusive breastfeeding for the first few months of life has been demonstrated to protect not only against various types of infection (respiratory, gastrointestinal, urinary, otitis media, and necrotising enterocolitis) [114, 115] but also against allergic diseases. For this reason, and others, breast milk is the ideal foodstuff for the newborn [116] as it provides the nutrients necessary for optimal growth and development. The composition of polyunsaturated fatty acids in breast milk is determined partly by the dietary PUFA content. There is a correlation between breast milk DHA levels and blood levels.

Likewise, there is a correlation between breast milk DHA levels and infant plasma levels [117, 118]. Other studies on supplementation have found a positive association between fish oil supplementation and a reduced plasma ω6/ω3 ratio in maternal plasma and in umbilical cord blood [119].

A dietary supply comprising mainly omega-6 fatty acids, as occurs in Western diets, can significantly inhibit the endogenous synthesis of omega-3 fatty acids, especially EPA and DHA given the enzymatic competition between their precursors. This becomes particularly relevant in the developing foetus and newborn, especially in premature or small-for-gestational-age babies [9]. Due to the limited capacity for synthesising these fatty acids [58], neonates are exclusively dependent on their placental transfer during pregnancy and their supply from breast milk. Therefore, a limited intake of omega-3 fatty acids in pregnancy or lactation can be associated with insufficient DHA levels for optimal neurological and immunological development in the foetus and newborn. In these states, a preventative nutritional intervention becomes particularly relevant as the fat that the mother consumes during pregnancy and lactation will greatly influence both foetal development and the lipid composition of breast milk and in turn the newborn's nutrition during the first stages of life [76, 120].

## 5. Patients and methods

We studied whether supplementing maternal diet with omega-3 LCPUFAs during the last trimester of pregnancy and the breastfeeding period influenced the levels of inflammatory cytokines in mother and child. Our study included a group of healthy infants born to term to 46 mothers, who had been enrolled in a registered, double-blind controlled randomised trial, from week 28 of pregnancy to the fourth month of lactation. Mothers were recruited in the Services of Gynecology of the Mother and Child Hospital of Granada, Spain (Hospital Materno-Infantil de Granada), and the Mother and Child University Hospital of Las Palmas de Gran Canaria, Spain (Complejo Hospitalario Universitario Insular Materno-Infantil de Canarias), between June 2009 and August 2010. Our sample was taken from an earlier larger study designed to assess the effects of omega-3 LCPUFA supplementation on the fatty acid profile of mothers and newborns [121]. The earlier study was registered on www.clinicaltrials.gov under identification code NCT01947426. The experimental groups were fish oil (FO) group ($n$ = 24) which received 400 ml of fish oil-enriched drink [320 mg DHA + 72 mg EPA] per day and control (CT) group ($n$ = 22) which received 400 ml of a non-supplemented drink per day. The dairy drinks were not commercially available products but specifically prepared for the study. The dietary supplementation started on week 28 of pregnancy and finished on the fourth month of lactation. We determined in mother and children plasma the concentrations of the following cytokines: GM-CSF, IL-2, IL-4, IL-6, IL-10, INF-γ, and TNF-α using MILLIPLEX® Human Cytokine/Chemokine kit in conjunction with a Luminex 200® system (Austin, TX, USA) and xPONENT® software package. The fatty acid profiles of maternal and children compartments were analysed in an earlier study [121], and DHA levels in mother and children plasma and erythrocyte membranes, as well as in breast milk, were used to evaluate correlation with cytokine levels.

## 6. Omega-3 fatty acids and cytokines during pregnancy

Supplementation with omega-3 LCPUFAs during pregnancy affects the pattern of fatty acids in maternal plasma and umbilical cord blood [122–124].

Supplementation increases DHA levels not only in these compartments but also in breast milk and in the infant's plasma if they are breastfed [121, 125].

Inflammation is considered one of the main causes of complications during pregnancy and of prematurity and neonatal morbidity [10–15]. Indeed, pregnancy may be considered a mild, controlled, systemic inflammatory state. Cytokines TNF-α and IL-1 are heavily involved in the inflammatory processes associated with pregnancy and labour [10, 12, 13], although an increase in inflammatory biomarkers such as IL-8, hepatocyte growth factor and monocyte chemotactic protein during pregnancy have also been demonstrated. There is also a progressive increase in vascular biomarkers, such as E-Selectin, vascular adhesion molecule 1, intercellular adhesion molecule (ICAM) 1, and plasminogen activator-inhibitor 1 [126]. Other studies have suggested that an abnormal response from cytokines and other molecules such as leptin may be involved in the pathophysiology of pregnancy-related complications such as preeclampsia. An association has been demonstrated between TNF-α, IL-6, IL-8, IL-10, and leptin, indicating that a rise in these markers could be used as a marker of inflammatory dysfunction and endothelial dysfunction in preeclampsia [103]. In women with a diagnosis of preeclampsia, increased levels of inflammatory cytokines such as IL-6 have even been found in breast milk [104].

Significant changes can also take place during pregnancy that affect lipid and carbohydrate metabolic pathways and vascular function. Adipose tissue acts as both a store of energy during pregnancy and a metabolically active tissue [126]. Adipocytes and their stroma are a rich source of cytokines and inflammatory mediators such as TNF-α and adiponectin, which increase and decrease insulin resistance, respectively [127]. The increased insulin resistance and the changes that occur in the maternal lipid profile during pregnancy could play an important role in endothelial dysfunction [128]. The role of adipokines, cytokines, and vascular homeostasis biomarkers in the regulation of metabolic changes during pregnancy remains to be fully established. There are a few studies, some of which are in animal models, that have investigated the effect on inflammation of omega-3 LCPUFA supplementation during pregnancy [34–36, 126, 129, 130].

A high intake of omega-3 fatty acids has been demonstrated to reduce the production of eicosanoids, cytokines, ROS and expression of adhesion molecules. Cell culture studies [33] have reported that EPA and DHA can inhibit the production of pro-inflammatory cytokines, such as TNF-α, IL-1, and IL-6, and in vitro studies have demonstrated that they can also reduce the expression of cell adhesion molecules and recently also in endothelial cells of the umbilical cord. These effects are supported by similar studies on dietary supplementation in animal and human models. In animal models, a reduction in the inflammatory response, expression of remodelling enzymes, and functional improvement has been demonstrated in offspring exposed to stressful situations whose mothers received DHA during pregnancy [34, 35]. In humans, some studies have revealed a decrease in cytokine levels, as a measure of systemic inflammatory response, after 8 weeks of fish oil supplementation [23]. During pregnancy, it has been demonstrated that intake of omega-3 long-chain fatty acids can modify cytokine levels and maturation of helper T (Th) cells [32]. Comparative studies in breastfed children whose mothers received EPA and DHA supplements from week 22 of pregnancy showed that this dietary intervention confers a reduction in Th1 cytokines such as IFN-gamma and IL-1 in the plasma and a reduction in the Th2 cytokines IL-14 and IL-13 in the umbilical cord blood [37]. In our study, in which mothers received supplements from week 28 of pregnancy and throughout breastfeeding, we found that levels of IL-6, TNF-α, IL-4, and IL-10 could be altered [26]. Maternal plasmatic levels of IL-10 and IL-4 were higher in the supplemental group (FO) than in the control group (CT). On the other hand, plasmatic IL-6 levels were higher both in mothers and children of the

CT group. Additionally, TNF-α was higher in CT children [26]. In a study on depression in pregnant women, it was also observed that prenatal EPA supplementation in particular reduced maternal levels of IL-6, Il-15, and TNF-α [131]. Clinically, these findings could translate to an increased anti-inflammatory "environment" provided by omega-3 LCPUFAs. TNF-α and IL-6 are pro-inflammatory, and IL-10, although it has both effects [131, 132], is considered the principal regulator of T cells and may act as an anti-inflammatory mediator of omega-3 LCPUFAs [133]. However, some studies have found no correlation between DHA and different cytokines: a study by Hawkes et al. [129] found that women receiving supplementation during pregnancy with a combination of 600 mg DHA plus 140 mg EPA daily for 4 weeks had an increase in omega-3 LCPUFA levels in the cells studied. DHA levels increased in a dose-dependent manner in the plasma and breast milk, which highlights the benefits of this dietary intervention. However, no significant differences were found between groups in the production of cytokines, either in breast milk cells or in peripheral blood. In addition to the dose, the duration of supplementation could be the key.

There has been some investigation into the clinical effect that supplementation may have on infants [133–136]. It has been observed that increased dietary intake of salmon during pregnancy increases levels of omega-3 LCPUFAs in umbilical cord plasma and affects cytokine production in neonates, with lower levels of IL-2, IL-4, IL-5, IL-10, and TNF-α in response to various stimuli [133]. Reduced IL-10 production has also been observed in vitro following stimulation with cat allergens in an atopic population [134]. Increased DHA and EPA in mother and child results in lower levels of PGE-2, a pro-inflammatory eicosanoid and inducer of IL-10 production, which could explain the reduced secretion of IL-10 in these individuals. This concept is also supported by Warstedt et al. [136] who suggested that reduced maternal levels of PGE-2 after omega-3 LCPUFA supplementation could contribute to a foetal immune system less prone to developing inflammatory disease such as allergies, since eicosanoids, cytokines, and chemokines are closely associated with the immune response. However, although results have been promising, it is still unclear whether or not omega-3 LCPUFAs affect the development of atopy [4].

Changes in fatty acid levels have been demonstrated to affect cytokine levels. A positive association has been observed between DHA and IL-10 such that at higher concentrations of DHA, IL-10 secretion is increased [26, 131]. Likewise, DHA has been negatively associated with IL-6, which could translate to an increased anti-inflammatory effect [26, 137]. These findings will need to be confirmed in future studies to clarify the uncertainties regarding the various mechanisms by which omega-3 LCPUFAs can affect inflammatory cytokines [137].

## 7. Conclusions

DHA supplementation during the third trimester of pregnancy and during breastfeeding can affect cytokine production, increasing anti-inflammatory cytokine levels and decreasing pro-inflammatory cytokine levels. These effects may translate to a lower risk of pregnancy-related complications and childhood disease, but much remains to be investigated in these fields.

## Acknowledgements

We thank all the members of our team who have participated in this work: Julio Ochoa, Federico Lara Villoslada, Naroa Kajarabille, Pedro Saavedra-Santana, Jose

Antonio Hurtado, Manuela Peña, Javier Diaz-Castro, Irma Sebastian-Garcia, Elisabet Machin-Martin, Magdalena Villanueva, Octavio Ramirez-Garcia, and NUGELA group. The authors have no financial relationships relevant to this chapter to disclose.

## Conflict of interest

The authors declare no conflict of interest.

## Author details

Yessica Rodriguez-Santana[1] and Luis Peña-Quintana[2,3,4*]

1 Primary Health Care "El Calero", Servicio Canario de Salud, Las Palmas, Spain

2 Unit of Pediatric Gastroenterology, Hepatology and Nutrition, Complejo Hospitalario Universitario Insular Materno-Infantil de Canarias, Las Palmas, Spain

3 Department of Clinical Sciences, University of Las Palmas de Gran Canaria, Spain

4 CIBER OBN, Spain

*Address all correspondence to: luis.pena@ulpgc.es

## References

[1] Larque E, Gil-Sanchez A, Prieto-Sanchez MT, Koletzko B. Omega 3 fatty acids, gestation and pregnancy outcomes. The British Journal of Nutrition. 2012;**107**(Suppl 2):S77-S84

[2] Helland IB, Smith L, Blomen B, Saarem K, Saugstad OD, Drevon CA. Effect of supplementing pregnant and lactating mothers with n-3 very-long-chain fatty acids on children's IQ and body mass index at 7 years of age. Pediatrics. 2008;**122**:e472-e479

[3] Gould JF, Smithers LG, Makrides M. The effect of maternal omega-3 (n-3) LCPUFA supplementation during pregnancy on early childhood cognitive and visual development: A systematic review and meta-analysis of randomized controlled trials. The American Journal of Clinical Nutrition. 2013;**97**:531-544

[4] De GR, Roggi C, Cena H. n-3 LC-PUFA supplementation: Effects on infant and maternal outcomes. European Journal of Nutrition. 2014;**53**:1147-1154

[5] Furuhjelm C, Warstedt K, Fageras M, Falth-Magnusson K, Larsson J, Fredriksson M, et al. Allergic disease in infants up to 2 years of age in relation to plasma omega-3 fatty acids and maternal fish oil supplementation in pregnancy and lactation. Pediatric Allergy and Immunology. 2011;**22**:505-514

[6] Dunstan JA, Mori TA, Barden A, Beilin LJ, Taylor AL, Holt PG, et al. Maternal fish oil supplementation in pregnancy reduces interleukin-13 levels in cord blood of infants at high risk of atopy. Clinical and Experimental Allergy. 2003;**33**:442-448

[7] Escamilla-Nunez MC, Barraza-Villarreal A, Hernandez-Cadena L, Navarro-Olivos E, Sly PD, Romieu I. Omega-3 fatty acid supplementation during pregnancy and respiratory symptoms in children. Chest. 2014;**146**:373-382

[8] Imhoff-Kunsch B, Stein AD, Martorell R, Parra-Cabrera S, Romieu I, Ramakrishnan U. Prenatal docosahexaenoic acid supplementation and infant morbidity: Randomized controlled trial. Pediatrics. 2011;**128**:e505-e512

[9] Rogers LK, Valentine CJ, Keim SA. DHA supplementation: Current implications in pregnancy and childhood. Pharmacological Research. 2013;**70**:13-19

[10] von Ehrenstein OS, Neta GI, Andrews W, Goldenberg R, Goepfert A, Zhang J. Child intellectual development in relation to cytokine levels in umbilical cord blood. American Journal of Epidemiology. 2012;**175**:1191-1199

[11] Yoon BH, Park CW, Chaiworapongsa T. Intrauterine infection and the development of cerebral palsy. BJOG. 2003;**110**(Suppl 20):124-127

[12] Pickler R, Brown L, McGrath J, Lyon D, Rattican D, Cheng CY, et al. Integrated review of cytokines in maternal, cord, and newborn blood: Part II—Associations with early infection and increased risk of neurologic damage in preterm infants. Biological Research for Nursing. 2010;**11**:377-386

[13] Pickler RH, McGrath JM, Reyna BA, McCain N, Lewis M, Cone S, et al. A model of neurodevelopmental risk and protection for preterm infants. The Journal of Perinatal & Neonatal Nursing. 2010;**24**:356-365

[14] Bland ST, Beckley JT, Young S, Tsang V, Watkins LR, Maier SF, et al. Enduring consequences of early-life

infection on glial and neural cell genesis within cognitive regions of the brain. Brain, Behavior, and Immunity. 2010;**24**:329-338

[15] Huleihel M, Golan H, Hallak M. Intrauterine infection/inflammation during pregnancy and offspring brain damages: Possible mechanisms involved. Reproductive Biology and Endocrinology. 2004;**2**:17

[16] Baldie G, Kaimakamis D, Rotondo D. Fatty acid modulation of cytokine release from human monocytic cells. Biochimica et Biophysica Acta. 1993;**1179**:125-133

[17] De CR, Cybulsky MI, Clinton SK, Gimbrone MA Jr, Libby P. The omega-3 fatty acid docosahexaenoate reduces cytokine-induced expression of proatherogenic and proinflammatory proteins in human endothelial cells. Arteriosclerosis and Thrombosis. 1994;**14**:1829-1836

[18] Khalfoun B, Thibault F, Watier H, Bardos P, Lebranchu Y. Docosahexaenoic and eicosapentaenoic acids inhibit in vitro human endothelial cell production of interleukin-6. Advances in Experimental Medicine and Biology. 1997;**400B**:589-597

[19] Chu AJ, Walton MA, Prasad JK, Seto A. Blockade by polyunsaturated n-3 fatty acids of endotoxin-induced monocytic tissue factor activation is mediated by the depressed receptor expression in THP-1 cells. The Journal of Surgical Research. 1999;**87**:217-224

[20] Endres S, Ghorbani R, Kelley VE, Georgilis K, Lonnemann G, van der Meer JW, et al. The effect of dietary supplementation with n-3 polyunsaturated fatty acids on the synthesis of interleukin-1 and tumor necrosis factor by mononuclear cells. The New England Journal of Medicine. 1989;**320**:265-271

[21] Meydani SN, Endres S, Woods MM, Goldin BR, Soo C, Morrill-Labrode A, et al. Oral (n-3) fatty acid supplementation suppresses cytokine production and lymphocyte proliferation: Comparison between young and older women. The Journal of Nutrition. 1991;**121**:547-555

[22] Gallai V, Sarchielli P, Trequattrini A, Franceschini M, Floridi A, Firenze C, et al. Cytokine secretion and eicosanoid production in the peripheral blood mononuclear cells of MS patients undergoing dietary supplementation with n-3 polyunsaturated fatty acids. Journal of Neuroimmunology. 1995;**56**:143-553

[23] Caughey GE, Mantzioris E, Gibson RA, Cleland LG, James MJ. The effect on human tumor necrosis factor alpha and interleukin 1 beta production of diets enriched in n-3 fatty acids from vegetable oil or fish oil. The American Journal of Clinical Nutrition. 1996;**63**:116-122

[24] Meydani SN, Lichtenstein AH, Cornwall S, Meydani M, Goldin BR, Rasmussen H, et al. Immunologic effects of national cholesterol education panel step-2 diets with and without fish-derived N-3 fatty acid enrichment. The Journal of Clinical Investigation. 1993;**92**:105-113

[25] Wachtler P, Konig W, Senkal M, Kemen M, Koller M. Influence of a total parenteral nutrition enriched with omega-3 fatty acids on leukotriene synthesis of peripheral leukocytes and systemic cytokine levels in patients with major surgery. The Journal of Trauma. 1997;**42**:191-198

[26] Rodriguez-Santana Y, Ochoa JJ, Lara-Villoslada F, Kajarabille N, Saavedra-Santana P, Hurtado JA, et al. Cytokine distribution in mothers and breastfed children after omega-3 LCPUFAs supplementation during the last trimester of pregnancy and

the lactation period: A randomized, controlled trial. Prostaglandins, Leukotrienes, and Essential Fatty Acids. 2017;**126**:32-38

[27] Miles EA, Calder PC. Influence of marine n-3 polyunsaturated fatty acids on immune function and a systematic review of their effects on clinical outcomes in rheumatoid arthritis. The British Journal of Nutrition. 2012;**107**(Suppl 2):S171-S184

[28] Dyall SC. Long-chain omega-3 fatty acids and the brain: A review of the independent and shared effects of EPA, DPA and DHA. Frontiers in Aging Neuroscience. 2015;7:52

[29] Serhan CN, Hong S, Gronert K, Colgan SP, Devchand PR, Mirick G, et al. Resolvins: A family of bioactive products of omega-3 fatty acid transformation circuits initiated by aspirin treatment that counter proinflammation signals. The Journal of Experimental Medicine. 2002;**196**:1025-1037

[30] Hong S, Gronert K, Devchand PR, Moussignac RL, Serhan CN. Novel docosatrienes and 17S-resolvins generated from docosahexaenoic acid in murine brain, human blood, and glial cells. Autacoids in anti-inflammation. The Journal of Biological Chemistry. 2003;**278**:14677-14687

[31] Uauy R, Mena P. Long-chain polyunsaturated fatty acids supplementation in preterm infants. Current Opinion in Pediatrics. 2015;**27**:165-171

[32] Lee HS, Barraza-Villarreal A, Hernandez-Vargas H, Sly PD, Biessy C, Ramakrishnan U, et al. Modulation of DNA methylation states and infant immune system by dietary supplementation with omega-3 PUFA during pregnancy in an intervention study. The American Journal of Clinical Nutrition. 2013;**98**:480-487

[33] Wang H, Khor TO, Saw CL, Lin W, Wu T, Huang Y, et al. Role of Nrf2 in suppressing LPS-induced inflammation in mouse peritoneal macrophages by polyunsaturated fatty acids docosahexaenoic acid and eicosapentaenoic acid. Molecular Pharmaceutics. 2010;7:2185-2193

[34] Rogers LK, Valentine CJ, Pennell M, Velten M, Britt RD, Dingess K, et al. Maternal docosahexaenoic acid supplementation decreases lung inflammation in hyperoxia-exposed newborn mice. The Journal of Nutrition. 2011;**141**(2):214-222

[35] Velten M, Britt RD Jr, Heyob KM, Tipple TE, Rogers LK. Maternal dietary docosahexaenoic acid supplementation attenuates fetal growth restriction and enhances pulmonary function in a newborn mouse model of perinatal inflammation. The Journal of Nutrition. 2014;**144**(3):258-266

[36] Ma L, Li N, Liu X, Shaw L, Li CS, Grant MB, et al. Arginyl-glutamine dipeptide or docosahexaenoic acid attenuate hyperoxia-induced lung injury in neonatal mice. Nutrition. 2012;**28**(11-12):1186-1191

[37] Granot E, Jakobovich E, Rabinowitz R, Levy P, Schlesinger M. DHA supplementation during pregnancy and lactation affects infants' cellular but not humoral immune response. Mediators of Inflammation. 2011;**2011**:493925

[38] Abedi E, Sahari MA. Long-chain polyunsaturated fatty acid sources and evaluation of their nutritional and functional properties. Food Science & Nutrition. 2014;**2**(5):443-463

[39] Doughman SD, Krupanidhi S, Sanjeevi CB. Omega-3 fatty acids for nutrition and medicine: Considering microalgae oil as a vegetarian source of EPA and DHA. Current Diabetes Reviews. 2007;**3**(3):198-203

[40] Williams CM, Burdge G. Long-chain n-3 PUFA: Plant v. marine sources. The Proceedings of the Nutrition Society. 2006;**65**(1):42-50

[41] Spector AA. Essentiality of fatty acids. Lipids. 1999;**34**(Suppl):S1-S3

[42] EFSA Panel on Dietetic Products NaAN. Scientific opinion on the tolerable upper intake level of eicosapentaenoic acid (EPA), docosahexaenoic acid (DHA) and docosapentaenoic acid (DPA). EFSA Journal. 2012;**10**:2815-2863. DOI: 10.2903/j.efsa.2012.2815. Available online: www.efsa.europa.eu/efsajourna

[43] Borges MC, Santos FM, Telles RW, Correia MI, Lanna CC. Polyunsaturated omega-3 fatty acids and systemic lupus erythematosus: What do we know? Revista Brasileira de Reumatologia. 2014;**54**(6):459-466

[44] Krauss RM, Eckel RH, Howard B, Appel LJ, Daniels SR, Deckelbaum RJ, et al. AHA dietary guidelines: Revision 2000: A statement for healthcare professionals from the nutrition Committee of the American Heart Association. Circulation. 2000;**102**(18):2284-2299

[45] Kris-Etherton PM, Harris WS, Appel LJ, American Heart Association. Nutrition Committee. Fish consumption, fish oil, omega-3 fatty acids, and cardiovascular disease. Circulation. 2002;**106**(21):2747-2757

[46] Hu FB, Bronner L, Willett WC, Stampfer MJ, Rexrode KM, Albert CM, et al. Fish and omega-3 fatty acid intake and risk of coronary heart disease in women. Journal of the American Medical Association. 2002;**287**(14):1815-1821

[47] Mozaffarian D, Ascherio A, Hu FB, Stampfer MJ, Willett WC, Siscovick DS, et al. Interplay between different polyunsaturated fatty acids and risk of coronary heart disease in men. Circulation. 2005;**111**(2):157-164

[48] Agostoni C, Bresson JL, Fairweather-Tait S, Flynn A, Golly I, Korhonen H, et al. Scientific opinion on the substantiation of health claims related to docosahexaenoic acid (DHA), eicosapentaenoic acid (EPA) and brain, eye and nerve development (ID 501, 513, 540), maintenance of normal brain function (ID 497, 501, 510, 513, 519, 521, 534, 540, 688, 1323, 1360, 4294), maintenance of normal vision (ID 508, 510, 513, 519, 529, 540, 688, 2905, 4294), maintenance of normal cardiac function (ID 510, 688, 1360), "maternal health; pregnancy and nursing" (ID 514), "to fulfill increased omega-3 fatty acids need during pregnancy" (ID 539), "skin and digestive tract epithelial cells maintenance" (ID 525), enhancement of mood (ID 536), "membranes cell structure" (ID 4295), "anti-inflammatory action" (ID 4688) and maintenance of normal blood LDLcholesterol concentrations (ID 4719) pursuant to article 13(1) of regulation (EC) No 1924/2006. EFSA Journal. 2011;9(40):2078. DOI: 10.2903/j.efsa.2011.2078. Available from: www.efsa.europa.eu/efsajournal

[49] Gorjao R, Azevedo-Martins AK, Rodrigues HG, Abdulkader F, Arcisio-Miranda M, Procopio J, et al. Comparative effects of DHA and EPA on cell function. Pharmacology & Therapeutics. 2009;**122**:56-64

[50] Onuki Y, Morishita M, Chiba Y, Tokiwa S, Takayama K. Docosahexaenoic acid and eicosapentaenoic acid induce changes in the physical properties of a lipid bilayer model membrane. Chemical & Pharmaceutical Bulletin (Tokyo). 2006;**54**:68-71

[51] Verlengia R, Gorjao R, Kanunfre CC, Bordin S, Martins De LT, Martins EF, et al. Comparative

effects of eicosapentaenoic acid and docosahexaenoic acid on proliferation, cytokine production, and pleiotropic gene expression in Jurkat cells. The Journal of Nutritional Biochemistry. 2004;**15**:657-665

[52] Holland D, Chang L, Ernst TM, Curran M, Buchthal SD, Alicata D, et al. Structural growth trajectories and rates of change in the first 3 months of infant brain development. JAMA Neurology. 2014;**71**:1266-1274

[53] Decsi T, Koletzko B. N-3 fatty acids and pregnancy outcomes. Current Opinion in Clinical Nutrition and Metabolic Care. 2005;**8**:161-166

[54] Koletzko B, Lien E, Agostoni C, Bohles H, Campoy C, Cetin I, et al. The roles of long-chain polyunsaturated fatty acids in pregnancy, lactation and infancy: Review of current knowledge and consensus recommendations. Journal of Perinatal Medicine. 2008;**36**:5-14

[55] Carlson SE, Werkman SH, Peeples JM, Wilson WM. Long-chain fatty acids and early visual and cognitive development of preterm infants. European Journal of Clinical Nutrition. 1994;**48**:S27-S30

[56] Bradbury J. Docosahexaenoic acid (DHA): An ancient nutrient for the modern human brain. Nutrients. 2011;**3**:529-554

[57] Innis SM. Perinatal biochemistry and physiology of long-chain polyunsaturated fatty acids. The Journal of Pediatrics. 2003;**143**:S1-S8

[58] Arterburn LM, Hall EB, Oken H. Distribution, interconversion, and dose response of n-3 fatty acids in humans. The American Journal of Clinical Nutrition. 2006;**83**:1467S-1476S

[59] Diau GY, Hsieh AT, Sarkadi-Nagy EA, Wijendran V, Nathanielsz PW, Brenna JT. The influence of long chain polyunsaturate supplementation on docosahexaenoic acid and arachidonic acid in baboon neonate central nervous system. BMC Medicine. 2005;**3**:11

[60] Favreliere S, Barrier L, Durand G, Chalon S, Tallineau C. Chronic dietary n-3 polyunsaturated fatty acids deficiency affects the fatty acid composition of plasmenylethanolamine and phosphatidylethanolamine differently in rat frontal cortex, striatum, and cerebellum. Lipids. 1998;**33**:401-407

[61] Bourre JM, Pascal G, Durand G, Masson M, Dumont O, Piciotti M. Alterations in the fatty acid composition of rat brain cells (neurons, astrocytes, and oligodendrocytes) and of subcellular fractions (myelin and synaptosomes) induced by a diet devoid of n-3 fatty acids. Journal of Neurochemistry. 1984;**43**:342-348

[62] Isaacs EB. Neuroimaging, a new tool for investigating the effects of early diet on cognitive and brain development. Frontiers in Human Neuroscience. 2013;**7**:445

[63] Meldrum SJ, D'Vaz N, Simmer K, Dunstan JA, Hird K, Prescott SL. Effects of high-dose fish oil supplementation during early infancy on neurodevelopment and language: A randomised controlled trial. The British Journal of Nutrition. 2012;**108**:1443-1454

[64] Colombo J, Carlson SE, Cheatham CL, Shaddy DJ, Kerling EH, Thodosoff JM, et al. Long-term effects of LCPUFA supplementation on childhood cognitive outcomes. The American Journal of Clinical Nutrition. 2013;**98**:403-412

[65] Drover J, Hoffman DR, Castaneda YS, Morale SE, Birch EE. Three randomized controlled trials of early long-chain polyunsaturated fatty acid supplementation on means-end

problem solving in 9-month-olds. Child Development. 2009;**80**:1376-1384

[66] Colombo J, Carlson SE, Cheatham CL, Fitzgerald-Gustafson KM, Kepler A, Doty T. Long-chain polyunsaturated fatty acid supplementation in infancy reduces heart rate and positively affects distribution of attention. Pediatric Research. 2011;**70**:406-410

[67] Drover JR, Hoffman DR, Castaneda YS, Morale SE, Garfield S, Wheaton DH, et al. Cognitive function in 18-month-old term infants of the DIAMOND study: A randomized, controlled clinical trial with multiple dietary levels of docosahexaenoic acid. Early Human Development. 2011;**87**:223-230

[68] Birch EE, Garfield S, Hoffman DR, Uauy R, Birch DG. A randomized controlled trial of early dietary supply of long-chain polyunsaturated fatty acids and mental development in term infants. Developmental Medicine and Child Neurology. 2000;**42**:174-181

[69] Willatts P, Forsyth S, Agostoni C, Casaer P, Riva E, Boehm G. Effects of long-chain PUFA supplementation in infant formula on cognitive function in later childhood. The American Journal of Clinical Nutrition. 2013;**98**:536S-542S

[70] Yavin E, Himovichi E, Eilam R. Delayed cell migration in the developing rat brain following maternal omega 3 alpha linolenic acid dietary deficiency. Neuroscience. 2009;**162**:1011-1022

[71] Calderon F, Kim HY. Docosahexaenoic acid promotes neurite growth in hippocampal neurons. Journal of Neurochemistry. 2004;**90**:979-988

[72] Ahmad A, Moriguchi T, Salem N. Decrease in neuron size in docosahexaenoic acid-deficient brain. Pediatric Neurology. 2002;**26**:210-218

[73] Cao D, Kevala K, Kim J, Moon HS, Jun SB, Lovinger D, et al. Docosahexaenoic acid promotes hippocampal neuronal development and synaptic function. Journal of Neurochemistry. 2009;**111**:510-521

[74] Vericel E, Colas R, Calzada C, Le QH, Feugier N, Cugnet C, et al. Moderate oral supplementation with docosahexaenoic acid improves platelet function and oxidative stress in type 2 diabetic patients. Thrombosis and Haemostasis. 2015;**114**:289-296

[75] Gil-Campos M, Dalmau SJ. Importance of docosahexaenoic acid (DHA): Functions and recommendations for its ingestion in infants. Anales de Pediatría (Barcelona, Spain). 2010;**73**:142-148

[76] Koletzko B, Cetin I, Brenna JT, The Perinatal Lipid Intake. Dietary fat intakes for pregnant and lactating women. The British Journal of Nutrition. 2007;**98**:873-877

[77] Ochoa JJ, Ramirez-Tortosa MC, Quiles JL, Palomino N, Robles R, Mataix J, et al. Oxidative stress in erythrocytes from premature and full-term infants during their first 72 h of life. Free Radical Research. 2003;**37**:317-322

[78] Ochoa JJ, Contreras-Chova F, Munoz S, Araujo-Nepomuceno E, Bonillo A, Molina-Carballo A, et al. Fluidity and oxidative stress in erythrocytes from very low birth weight infants during their first 7 days of life. Free Radical Research. 2007;**41**:1035-1040

[79] Garrel C, Alessandri JM, Guesnet P, Al-Gubory KH. Omega-3 fatty acids enhance mitochondrial superoxide dismutase activity in rat organs during post-natal development. The International Journal of Biochemistry & Cell Biology. 2012;**44**:123-131

[80] Garcia-Rodriguez CE, Mesa MD, Olza J, Vlachava M, Kremmyda LS, Diaper ND, et al. Does consumption of two portions of salmon per

week enhance the antioxidant defense system in pregnant women? Antioxidants & Redox Signaling. 2012;**16**:1401-1406

[81] Calder PC. Polyunsaturated fatty acids and inflammation. Prostaglandins, Leukotrienes, and Essential Fatty Acids. 2006;**75**:197-202

[82] Moghaddami M, James M, Proudman S, Cleland LG. Synovial fluid and plasma n3 long chain polyunsaturated fatty acids in patients with inflammatory arthritis. Prostaglandins, Leukotrienes, and Essential Fatty Acids. 2015;**97**:7-12

[83] McKarney C, Everard M, N'Diaye T. Omega-3 fatty acids (from fish oils) for cystic fibrosis. Cochrane Database of Systematic Reviews. 2007;**4**:CD002201

[84] Farinotti M, Vacchi L, Simi S, Di PC, Brait L, Filippini G. Dietary interventions for multiple sclerosis. Cochrane Database of Systematic Reviews. 2012;**12**:CD004192

[85] Farinotti M, Simi S, Di PC, McDowell N, Brait L, Lupo D, et al. Dietary interventions for multiple sclerosis. Cochrane Database of Systematic Reviews. 2007;**1**:CD004192

[86] Grimstad T, Berge RK, Bohov P, Skorve J, Goransson L, Omdal R, et al. Salmon diet in patients with active ulcerative colitis reduced the simple clinical colitis activity index and increased the anti-inflammatory fatty acid index—A pilot study. Scandinavian Journal of Clinical and Laboratory Investigation. 2011;**71**:68-73

[87] Hartweg J, Perera R, Montori V, Dinneen S, Neil HA, Farmer A. Omega-3 polyunsaturated fatty acids (PUFA) for type 2 diabetes mellitus. Cochrane Database of Systematic Reviews. 2008;**1**:CD003205

[88] Ellulu MS, Khaza'ai H, Abed Y, Rahmat A, Ismail P, Ranneh Y. Role of fish oil in human health and possible mechanism to reduce the inflammation. Inflammopharmacology. 2015;**23**:79-89

[89] Carrero JJ, Martin-Bautista E, Baro L, Fonolla J, Jimenez J, Boza JJ, et al. Cardiovascular effects of omega-3-fatty acids and alternatives to increase their intake. Nutrición Hospitalaria. 2005;**20**:63-69

[90] Pirillo A, Catapano AL. Update on the management of severe hypertriglyceridemia—Focus on free fatty acid forms of omega-3. Drug Design, Development and Therapy. 2015;**9**:2129-2137

[91] Harris WS, Dayspring TD, Moran TJ. Omega-3 fatty acids and cardiovascular disease: New developments and applications. Postgraduate Medicine. 2013;**125**:100-113

[92] Weintraub H. Update on marine omega-3 fatty acids: Management of dyslipidemia and current omega-3 treatment options. Atherosclerosis. 2013;**230**:381-389

[93] Weintraub HS. Overview of prescription omega-3 fatty acid products for hypertriglyceridemia. Postgraduate Medicine. 2014;**126**:7-18

[94] Carrero JJ, Grimble RF. Does nutrition have a role in peripheral vascular disease? The British Journal of Nutrition. 2006;**95**:217-229

[95] Calder PC. n-3 fatty acids and cardiovascular disease: Evidence explained and mechanisms explored. Clinical Science (London, England). 2004;**107**:1-11

[96] Mocellin MC, Camargo CQ, Nunes EA, Fiates GM, Trindade EB. A systematic review and meta-analysis of the n-3 polyunsaturated fatty acids effects on inflammatory markers in colorectal cancer. Clinical Nutrition. 2015;**29**:123-125

[97] de Aguiar Pastore SJ, Emilia de Souza FM, Waitzberg DL. Omega-3 supplements for patients in chemotherapy and/or radiotherapy: A systematic review. Clinical Nutrition. 2015;**34**:359-366

[98] Laviano A, Rianda S, Molfino A, Rossi FF. Omega-3 fatty acids in cancer. Current Opinion in Clinical Nutrition and Metabolic Care. 2013;**16**:156-161

[99] Merendino N, Costantini L, Manzi L, Molinari R, D'Eliseo D, Velotti F. Dietary omega-3 polyunsaturated fatty acid DHA: A potential adjuvant in the treatment of cancer. BioMed Research International. 2013;**2013**:310186. DOI: 10.1155/2013/310186

[100] Jing K, Wu T, Lim K. Omega-3 polyunsaturated fatty acids and cancer. Anti-Cancer Agents in Medicinal Chemistry. 2013;**13**:1162-1177

[101] Calder PC. n-3 polyunsaturated fatty acids, inflammation, and inflammatory diseases. The American Journal of Clinical Nutrition. 2006;**83**:1505S-1519S

[102] Schaue D, Kachikwu EL, McBride WH. Cytokines in radiobiological responses: A review. Radiation Research. 2012;**178**:505-523

[103] Sharma A, Satyam A, Leptin SJB. IL-10 and inflammatory markers (TNF-alpha, IL-6 and IL-8) in pre-eclamptic, normotensive pregnant and healthy non-pregnant women. American Journal of Reproductive Immunology. 2007;**58**:21-30

[104] Freitas NA, Santiago LTC, Kurokawa CS, Meira Junior JD, Corrente JE, Rugolo LMSS. Effect of preeclampsia on human milk cytokine levels. The Journal of Maternal-Fetal & Neonatal Medicine. 2018;**25**:1-5. DOI: 10.1080/14767058.2018.1429395

[105] Murphy AM, Lyons CL, Finucane OM, Roche HM. Interactions between differential fatty acid and inflammatory stressors-impact on metabolic health. Prostaglandins, Leukotrienes, and Essential Fatty Acids. 2015;**92**:49-55

[106] Giorlandino C, Giannarelli D. Effect of vaginally administered DHA fatty acids on pregnancy outcome in high risk pregnancies for preterm delivery: A double blinded randomised controlled trial. Journal of Prenatal Medicine. 2013;**7**:42-45

[107] Otto SJ, van Houwelingen AC, Badart-Smook A, Hornstra G. Comparison of the peripartum and postpartum phospholipid polyunsaturated fatty acid profiles of lactating and nonlactating women. The American Journal of Clinical Nutrition. 2001;**73**:1074-1079

[108] Lauritzen L, Carlson SE. Maternal fatty acid status during pregnancy and lactation and relation to newborn and infant status. Maternal & Child Nutrition. 2011;**7**:41-58

[109] Berghaus TM, Demmelmair H, Koletzko B. Essential fatty acids and their long-chain polyunsaturated metabolites in maternal and cord plasma triglycerides during late gestation. Biology of the Neonate. 2000;**77**:96-100

[110] Su HM. Mechanisms of n-3 fatty acid-mediated development and maintenance of learning memory performance. The Journal of Nutritional Biochemistry. 2010;**21**:364-373

[111] Decsi T, Campoy C, Koletzko B. Effect of N-3 polyunsaturated fatty acid supplementation in pregnancy: The Nuheal trial. Advances in Experimental Medicine and Biology. 2005;**569**:109-113

[112] Hawkes JS, Bryan DL, James MJ, Gibson RA. Cytokines (IL-1beta, IL-6, TNF-alpha, TGF-beta1, and TGF-beta2) and prostaglandin E2 in human milk during the first three

months postpartum. Pediatric Research. 1999;**46**:194-199

[113] Urwin HJ, Miles EA, Noakes PS, Kremmyda LS, Vlachava M, Diaper ND, et al. Salmon consumption during pregnancy alters fatty acid composition and secretory IgA concentration in human breast milk. The Journal of Nutrition. 2012;**142**:1603-1610

[114] Beaudry M, Dufour R, Marcoux S. Relation between infant feeding and infections during the first six months of life. The Journal of Pediatrics. 1995;**126**:191-197

[115] Hanson LA. Human milk and host defence: Immediate and long-term effects. Acta Paediatrica. Supplement. 1999;**88**:42-46

[116] Koletzko B, Boey CC, Campoy C, Carlson SE, Chang N, Guillermo-Tuazon MA, et al. Current information and Asian perspectives on long-chain polyunsaturated fatty acids in pregnancy, lactation, and infancy: Systematic review and practice recommendations from an early nutrition academy workshop. Annals of Nutrition & Metabolism. 2014;**65**(1):49-80

[117] Jensen CL, Maude M, Anderson RE, Heird WC. Effect of docosahexaenoic acid supplementation of lactating women on the fatty acid composition of breast milk lipids and maternal and infant plasma phospholipids. The American Journal of Clinical Nutrition. 2000;**71**:292S-299S

[118] Escolano-Margarit MV, Campoy C, Ramirez-Tortosa MC, Demmelmair H, Miranda MT, Gil A, et al. Effects of fish oil supplementation on the fatty acid profile in erythrocyte membrane and plasma phospholipids of pregnant women and their offspring: A randomised controlled trial. The British Journal of Nutrition. 2013;**109**:1647-1656

[119] Much D, Brunner S, Vollhardt C, Schmid D, Sedlmeier EM, Bruderl M, et al. Effect of dietary intervention to reduce the n-6/n-3 fatty acid ratio on maternal and fetal fatty acid profile and its relation to offspring growth and body composition at 1 year of age. European Journal of Clinical Nutrition. 2013;**67**:282-288

[120] Christian P. Maternal nutrition, health, and survival. Nutrition Reviews. 2002;**60**:S59-S63

[121] Hurtado JA, Iznaola C, Pena M, Ruiz J, Pena-Quintana L, Kajarabille N, et al. Effects of maternal Omega-3 supplementation on fatty acids and on visual and cognitive development: A randomized trial. Journal of Pediatric Gastroenterology and Nutrition. 2015;**61**:472-480. DOI: 10.1097/MPG.0000000000000864

[122] van Houwelingen AC, Sorensen JD, Hornstra G, Simonis MM, Boris J, Olsen SF, et al. Essential fatty acid status in neonates after fish-oil supplementation during late pregnancy. The British Journal of Nutrition. 1995;**74**:723-731

[123] Al MD, von Houwelingen AC, Badart-Smook A, Hornstra G. Some aspects of neonatal essential fatty acid status are altered by linoleic acid supplementation of women during pregnancy. The Journal of Nutrition. 1995;**125**:2822-2830

[124] Krauss-Etschmann S, Shadid R, Campoy C, Hoster E, Demmelmair H, Jimenez M, et al. Effects of fish-oil and folate supplementation of pregnant women on maternal and fetal plasma concentrations of docosahexaenoic acid and eicosapentaenoic acid: A European randomized multicenter trial. The American Journal of Clinical Nutrition. 2007;**85**:1392-1400

[125] Helland IB, Saugstad OD, Saarem K, van Houwelingen AC, Nylander G, Drevon CA. Supplementation of n-3

fatty acids during pregnancy and lactation reduces maternal plasma lipid levels and provides DHA to the infants. The Journal of Maternal-Fetal & Neonatal Medicine. 2006;**19**:397-406

[126] Garcia-Rodriguez CE, Olza J, Aguilera CM, Mesa MD, Miles EA, Noakes PS, et al. Plasma inflammatory and vascular homeostasis biomarkers increase during human pregnancy but are not affected by oily fish intake. The Journal of Nutrition. 2012;**142**:1191-1196

[127] Briana DD, Malamitsi-Puchner A. Reviews: Adipocytokines in normal and complicated pregnancies. Reproductive Sciences. 2009;**16**:921-937

[128] Paradisi G, Biaggi A, Ferrazzani S, De CS, Caruso A. Abnormal carbohydrate metabolism during pregnancy: Association with endothelial dysfunction. Diabetes Care. 2002;**25**:560-564

[129] Hawkes JS, Bryan DL, Makrides M, Neumann MA, Gibson RA. A randomized trial of supplementation with docosahexaenoic acid-rich tuna oil and its effects on the human milk cytokines interleukin 1 beta, interleukin 6, and tumor necrosis factor alpha. The American Journal of Clinical Nutrition. 2002;**75**:754-760

[130] Frew L, Sugiarto NU, Rajagopal SP, He J, Leask R, Norman JE, et al. The effect of omega-3 polyunsaturated fatty acids on the inflammatory response of the amnion. Prostaglandins, Leukotrienes, and Essential Fatty Acids. 2013;**89**:221-225

[131] Mozurkewich EL, Berman DR, Vahratian A, Clinton CM, Romero VC, Chilimigras JL, et al. Effect of prenatal EPA and DHA on maternal and umbilical cord blood cytokines. BMC Pregnancy and Childbirth. 2018;**18**: 261-269. DOI: 10.1186/s12884-018-1899-6

[132] Mannino MH, Zhu Z, Xiao H, Bai Q, Wakefield MR, Fang Y. The paradoxical role of IL-10 in immunity and cancer. Cancer Letters. 2015;**367**:103-107

[133] Noakes PS, Vlachava M, Kremmyda LS, Diaper ND, Miles EA, Erlewyn-Lajeunesse M, et al. Increased intake of oily fish in pregnancy: Effects on neonatal immune responses and on clinical outcomes in infants at 6 mo. The American Journal of Clinical Nutrition. 2012;**95**:395-404

[134] Dunstan JA, Mori TA, Barden A, Beilin LJ, Taylor AL, Holt PG, et al. Fish oil supplementation in pregnancy modifies neonatal allergen-specific immune responses and clinical outcomes in infants at high risk of atopy: A randomized, controlled trial. The Journal of Allergy and Clinical Immunology. 2003;**112**:1178-1184

[135] Chase HP, Boulware D, Rodriguez H, Donaldson D, Chritton S, Rafkin-Mervis L, et al. Effect of docosahexaenoic acid supplementation on inflammatory cytokine levels in infants at high genetic risk for type 1 diabetes. Pediatric Diabetes. 2015;**16**:271-279

[136] Warstedt K, Furuhjelm C, Duchen K, Falth-Magnusson K, Fageras M. The effects of omega-3 fatty acid supplementation in pregnancy on maternal eicosanoid, cytokine, and chemokine secretion. Pediatric Research. 2009;**66**:212-217

[137] Vedin I, Cederholm T, Freund LY, Basun H, Garlind A, Faxen IG, et al. Effects of docosahexaenoic acid-rich n-3 fatty acid supplementation on cytokine release from blood mononuclear leukocytes: The OmegAD study. The American Journal of Clinical Nutrition. 2008;**87**:1616-1622

Chapter 4

# Correlates of Caesarean Section Delivery in West Bengal, India: An Analysis Based on DLHS-3

*Rayhan SK and Somdutta Barua*


## Abstract

It has been well recognised that medically unnecessary caesarean section (C-section) delivery could increase morbidity risks for both the mother and her child and also could put strain on both institutional and individual assets mainly in developing countries. The present study tried to assess the variations in C-section delivery rates by women's background characteristics and to examine the factors associated with C-section delivery in West Bengal—a state of India. Data from the third round of the District Level Household and Facility Survey (DLHS-3) 2007–2008, covering 6447 ever-married women of age 15–49 years, were used. The results reveal that about 12% women delivered their babies by C-section irrespective of place of delivery, but it rose to about 24% in only institutional delivery. It is also found that the rate of C-section delivery was excessively high in private health facilities (55.8%) followed by higher educated women (50.4%) and for health insurance (36.4%), and antenatal care service eight or more times (36%). The results of predicted (adjusted) probability computed from logistic regression reveal that delivery in private health facilities, higher maternal age, lower birth order and higher level of education were the main influential factors of C-section delivery.


**Keywords:** antenatal care (ANC), place of delivery, caesarean section delivery, West Bengal, India

## 1. Introduction

The operation for caesarean delivery constitutes a major surgical procedure. There are a large number of adverse effects on women and infants after the C-section delivery. Study found that C-section delivery is associated with a higher risk of ureteral tract and vesical damage, hysterectomy, abdominal pain, maternal mortality, uterine rupture in future pregnancies, neonatal respiratory morbidity, placenta previa and foetal death [1]. It was revealed that women who delivered their baby by elective C-section have 2.84 times more chance of maternal death than women who delivered their baby normally [2]. A study from Africa found that C-section delivery is associated with stillbirths, neonatal deaths and neonatal morbidity [3]. C-section delivery individually minimises the overall risk to foetus death from the breech birth presentations, although it raises the risk of severe neonatal and maternal morbidities and mortality in cephalic presentation [4]. Women who delivered their first baby by C-section have slightly higher long-term morbidity



IntechOpen

than those women delivered their baby normally [5]. A study from Mexico revealed that children born by C-section are less likely to receive breastfeeding than the children born normally [6]. There is also evidence from highly developed countries that C-section is associated with adverse psychosocial results, for example, dissatisfaction, distress and problem with woman and child bonding [7]. Another study demonstrated that caesarean childbirths lead to higher financial burden than vaginal deliveries [8].

In this regard, the World Health Organization (WHO) issued an agreement proclamation in 1985, stating that, "There is no justification for any region to have C-section (CS) rates higher than 10–15%" [9]. But there is considerable debate about whether CS rates over 15% mean an over-utilisation of the procedure. But it is true that "as with any surgery, caesarean sections are associated with short and long term risk which can extend many years beyond the current delivery and affect the health of the woman, her child, and future pregnancies. These risks are higher in women with limited access to comprehensive obstetric care" [10]. According to the District Level Household and Facility Survey (DLHS), the average C-section rate in West Bengal was 11.8% in DLHS-3, 2007–2008 [11], and it also varied from district to district in West Bengal. There was interdistrict variation in C-section rates in West Bengal with Kolkata having the highest C-section rate (34.1%), and Malda having the lowest C-section rate (only 1.8%) in DLHS-3, 2007–2008 [11]. The rate of C-section increased significantly from 3.4% in DLHS-2, 2002–2004 [12], to about 12% in DLHS-3, 2007–2008, and again it rose to 22% (Factsheet DLHS-3, 2012–2013) [13], which was a matter of concern.

The present study was based on the following four observations which were conceptualised by Leone et al. [14]: *first*, recent increasing trends in C-section delivery in West Bengal; *second*, evidence that medically unnecessary C-section could increase morbidity risks for both the woman and her child; *third*, unnecessary medical interventions and C-section could put strain on both institutional and individual assets; *fourth*, evidence from more developed countries demonstrates that C-section delivery is associated with adverse psychosocial outcomes such as distress, dissatisfaction and problems with maternal-infant bonding. On the basis of these observations, the present study tried to explore variations in C-section delivery rates by women's background characteristics and to examine the factors influencing the C-section delivery in West Bengal—a state of Eastern India. The findings of this study could be helpful for policymakers and planning to improve women's health and to make appropriate use of healthcare resources.

This study surveyed the existing studies and tried to find out the associated non-clinical factors of C-section delivery for selecting the relevant independent factors for the present analysis. Among maternal factors, previous studies found that the probability of having C-section delivery increases with the increase in maternal age [15–18]; the likelihood of having C-section delivery decreases with the increase in parity [19–21]. Among socioeconomic factors, existing studies showed that the probability of having C-section delivery increases with the increase in the maternal level of education [16, 22, 23]; with the increase in the level of income, the probability of having C-section delivery also increases [24, 25]; urban women tend to have more C-section delivery than rural women [26, 27]. Among institutional factors, previous studies found that the type of hospitals and number of antenatal care (ANC) visits play a vital role for C-section delivery. Delivering in private health facilities has higher tendency to undergo C-section delivery than delivering in public hospitals [20, 28–31]. The likelihood of C-section delivery increases with the increase in number of ANC visits [19, 21, 32]. Women who have health insurance are more likely to have C-section delivery than women who do not have any health insurance [33, 34].

## 2. Data and methods

The present analysis was based on the data from the third round of the District Level Household and Facility Survey, carried out during December 2007–2008 in India (DLHS-3, 2007–2008). The District Level Household and Facility Survey was a countywide survey covering 601 districts of India [11]. This survey was designed to gather information at the district level on different aspects of women's healthcare utilisation for Reproductive and Child Health (RCH) including accessibility to the health facilities and to evaluate the health facility capacity and readiness regarding infrastructure. DLHS-3 surveyed a sum of 22213 households and 21878 ever-married women in West Bengal. However, this study was based on 6447 ever-married women of age 15–49 years who had given live birth between January 1, 2004, and the survey date. This was the third round of data which were in the public domain.

### 2.1 Outcome variable

The outcome or dependent variable was C-section delivery; a dichotomous variable was coded as "1" for yes and "0" for no, or, simply, those women aged 15–49 years who delivered their last live birth after January 1, 2004, by surgical procedure were coded as "1", and those women aged 15–49 years who delivered their last live birth after January 1, 2004, by natural process/vaginally or with assistance or instrument were coded as "0".

### 2.2 Explanatory variables

The C-section delivery is an outcome of demographic, socioeconomic, insurance status and institutional factors. Among demographic factors, maternal age at last birth (below 20, 20–24, 25–29 and 30+ years) and birth order (first birth order, second birth order and third birth order or above) were taken. The level of mother's education (no schooling, up to 5 years, 6–10 years, 11+ years), household wealth index (poor, middle and rich), religion (Hindus, Muslims and others), caste/tribe (Scheduled Caste (SC), Scheduled Tribe (ST) and others or general) and place of residences (rural and urban residence) were taken from socioeconomic factors. Coverage by health insurance scheme (yes, no) was also included as an explanatory variable. Antenatal care services include the number of ANC visits (up to three times, four to seven times and eight or more times) and places of ANC services (no ANC visits, only public health facilities, only private health facilities, public/private health facilities, and home or elsewhere), and the place of delivery (public health facilities, private health facilities) were taken from institutional factors.

### 2.3 Statistical analysis

The differences in C-section delivery by women's background characteristics were gross differentials and had been obtained through bivariate analysis. As a number of factors were strongly associated with each other, there was the possibility of confounding. Therefore, it was necessarily desirable to detect the net effect. For this purpose, logistic regression model had been used. In this model, the coefficient (B) and odds ratio (Exp B) were estimated. In order to assess the true differences, it was desirable to obtain adjusted probabilities; by that one can see the actual difference in probabilities [35]. The adjusted probabilities were computed from the coefficients of logistic regression analysis for C-section delivery. A p-value of less than and equal to 0.05 was considered as the significant association between independent variable and outcome variable.

## 3. Results

**Table 1** presents the results of bivariate analysis of C-section delivery rates, by the place of delivery, among all deliveries and all institutional deliveries by the women's background characteristics. From **Table 1**, it was found that among all deliveries, about 12% of women delivered their last birth by C-section, while it was about 24% among all institutional deliveries. And by place of delivery, it was 58.8 and 15.2% for private and public hospitals, respectively. Among all deliveries, it was observed that the proportion of C-section delivery increased with the increases in the maternal age, while the rate of C-section delivery decreased with the increases in birth order. With an increase in the number of ANC visits, the proportion of C-section delivery also increased. The proportions of C-section delivery were higher for receiving ANC services at only private hospitals and for receiving ANC services at both the private and public hospitals than the categories of not receiving any ANC services, receiving it at home and receiving it at public hospitals only. With the increase in the mother's level of education and household's income, the rates of C-section delivery also increased. The percent of C-section delivery was relatively higher for Hindus than that of Muslims and other minor religious groups. Also, the rate of C-section delivery was higher for other categories (general or non-deprived population) than the deprived communities, that is, Scheduled Caste (SC) and Scheduled Tribe (ST). As compared with rural areas, C-section delivery rate was higher for urban areas. Further, the rate of C-section delivery was quite higher for the women who had health insurance than those who had not. However, the rate of C-section delivery was excessively high for the women who delivered their babies in private health facilities (55.8%) followed by the women who attained higher secondary or more education (50.4%), women who had health insurance (36.4%), women who had received antenatal care service eight or more times (36%), women who had received ANC service in only private health facilities (30.4%) and women who lived in urban areas (29.7%). Besides, women who had only one child, received ANC service four to seven times, received ANC service in both public health facilities and private health facilities, attained upper primary or secondary education and delivered their infants in public health facilities present above 15% of C-section delivery rate in West Bengal. On the other hand, the rates of caesarean delivery were very low, which was lower than 5% for the women who had three children, women who did not receive any ANC service, women who received ANC service at home or elsewhere, illiterate women, poor women and tribal women.

**Table 2** presents the results of the logistic regression analysis and adjusted probabilities which were computed from the coefficients of logistic regression analysis for C-section delivery. The logistic regression analysis included only the women (unweighted no. = 3149) of age 15–49 years who had given live birth in any health facilities since January 1, 2004, in West Bengal because performing of C-section is possible only in health institutions. Women's background characteristics, utilisation of antenatal care and delivery care service were considered as independent variables, and the type of delivery (normal delivery or C-section delivery) was taken as a dependent variable in this analysis. The actual probability of C-section delivery was 24.1% (weighted) for all the women who had given live birth in any health facilities. The results showed that the place of delivery and number of ANC visits were the significant factors of C-section delivery among institutional factors; maternal age and birth order were the significant factors of C-section delivery among demographic factors; and the level of maternal education was the only one factor significantly associated with the C-section delivery among socioeconomic factors. Delivery in private health facility was the strongest predictor of C-section delivery after controlling for other variables. The adjusted probability of having

| Background characteristics | C-section delivery rate (%) | | | | | Number of women | |
|---|---|---|---|---|---|---|---|
| | Place of delivery | | | All deliveries | All institutional deliveries | Weighted | Unweighted |
| | Public # | Private # | Home/ elsewhere | | | | |
| **Age** | | | | | | | |
| <20 years | 11.5 | 43.8 | 0 | **8.4** | **16** | 1756 | 1759 |
| 20–24 years | 15.9 | 56.4 | 0 | **12.5** | **24.9** | 2723 | 2727 |
| 25–29 years | 18 | 62.1 | 0 | **14.3** | **30.3** | 1321 | 1323 |
| 30+ years | 21.5 | 58.8 | 0 | **13.3** | **34.3** | 637 | 638 |
| **Birth order** | | | | | | | |
| 1 | 18.9 | 57.4 | 0 | **19.6** | **28.5** | 2505 | 2502 |
| 2 | 13.3 | 57.7 | 0 | **10.5** | **22.4** | 2029 | 2029 |
| 3+ | 7.5 | 39.7 | 0 | **3.1** | **12** | 1904 | 1916 |
| **No. of ANC visits** | | | | | | | |
| Up to 3 times | 11.4 | 43.6 | 0 | **5.3** | **15.4** | 3640 | 3658 |
| 4–7 times | 16.6 | 55 | 0 | **16.7** | **26.1** | 2281 | 2278 |
| 8+ times | 25.2 | 68.4 | 0 | **36** | **42.8** | 517 | 511 |
| **Place of ANC visits** | | | | | | | |
| No ANC visits | 22.9 | 0 | 0 | **3.1** | **20** | 258 | 259 |
| Only public # | 12.3 | 47 | 0 | **6** | **14.5** | 3675 | 3687 |
| Only private # | 22.8 | 57.3 | 0 | **30.4** | **41.4** | 970 | 967 |
| Public/private # | 17.5 | 58.4 | 0 | **17** | **27.1** | 1369 | 1368 |
| Home/elsewhere | 12 | 66.7 | 0 | **3** | **17.9** | 167 | 166 |
| **Education** | | | | | | | |
| No schooling | 10.6 | 32.2 | 0 | **3.7** | **12.6** | 2218 | 2236 |
| Up to 5 years | 12.1 | 42.2 | 0 | **6.7** | **15.9** | 1696 | 1701 |
| 6–10 years | 16.3 | 54.7 | 0 | **16.9** | **25.4** | 2105 | 2094 |
| 11+ years | 35.4 | 69.7 | 0 | **50.2** | **54** | 419 | 416 |
| **Income (wealth index)** | | | | | | | |
| Poor | 9.6 | 58.5 | 0 | **3.8** | **13.2** | 1929 | 1945 |
| Middle | 11.8 | 44.1 | 0 | **6.8** | **15.7** | 2776 | 2779 |
| Rich | 22.4 | 59 | 0 | **28.9** | **35.6** | 1733 | 1723 |
| **Religion group** | | | | | | | |
| Muslims | 15.9 | 45.5 | 0 | **6.9** | **20.9** | 1976 | 1988 |
| Hindus | 15 | 57.9 | 0 | **14.1** | **24.9** | 4368 | 4365 |
| Others | 19.2 | 37.5 | 0 | **8.6** | **23.5** | 93 | 94 |
| **Social group** | | | | | | | |
| Scheduled Caste | 12 | 50.4 | 0 | **8.2** | **17.1** | 1953 | 1964 |
| Scheduled Tribe | 11.3 | 41.2 | 0 | **4.4** | **14.3** | 545 | 548 |
| Others | 17.4 | 57.5 | 0 | **14.7** | **28.1** | 3940 | 3935 |
| **Place of residence** | | | | | | | |
| Rural | 12.4 | 54.9 | 0 | **8.7** | **20** | 5466 | 5474 |
| Urban | 25.5 | 57.4 | 0 | **29.7** | **36.4** | 972 | 973 |

| Background characteristics | C-section delivery rate (%) | | | | | Number of women | |
|---|---|---|---|---|---|---|---|
| | Place of delivery | | | All deliveries | All institutional deliveries | Weighted | Unweighted |
| | Public # | Private # | Home/ elsewhere | | | | |
| **Insurance coverage** | | | | | | | |
| No | 14.9 | 55.2 | 0 | **11.1** | **23.1** | 6254 | 6263 |
| Yes | 29 | 61 | 0 | **36.4** | **45.9** | 184 | 184 |
| **All** | **15.2** | **55.8** | **0** | **11.8** | **24.1** | **6438** | **6447** |

*Note: # = type of health facilities*
*Sources: Computed from DLHS-3 data files.*

**Table 1.**
*C-section delivery rates by women's background characteristics, antenatal care service and place of delivery in West Bengal, DLHS-3, 2007–2008.*

| Background characteristics | No. of women | B | Odds ratio | Unadjusted probabilities (in percent) | Predicted probabilities (in percent) |
|---|---|---|---|---|---|
| *Institutional factors* | | | | | |
| **Place of delivery** | | | | | |
| Public health facilities® | 2460 | 0 | 0 | 15.2 | 18.3 |
| Private health facilities | 689 | 1.4839 | 4.4*** | 55.8 | 49.6*** |
| **Place of ANC services** | | | | | |
| No ANC visits® | 40 | 0 | 0 | 20 | 32.6 |
| Only public health facilities | 1516 | −0.577 | 0.5767 | 14.5 | 21.6 |
| Only private health facilities | 709 | −0.399 | 0.68 | 41.4 | 24.8 |
| Public and private | 856 | −0.323 | 0.724 | 27.1 | 26 |
| Home/elsewhere | 28 | −0.31 | 0.734 | 17.9 | 26.2 |
| **No. of ANC visits** | | | | | |
| Up to 3 times® | 1260 | 0 | 0 | 15.4 | 21.1 |
| 4–8 times | 1459 | 0.1878 | 1.194 | 26.1 | 24.2 |
| 8+ times | 430 | 0.4545 | 1.6** | 42.8 | 29.5** |
| *Demographic factors* | | | | | |
| **Age** | | | | | |
| <20 years® | 921 | 0 | 0 | 16 | 16.7 |
| 20–24 years | 1363 | 0.4766 | 1.6*** | 24.9 | 24.2*** |
| 25–29 years | 620 | 0.8215 | 2.3*** | 30.3 | 31.1*** |
| 30+ years | 245 | 0.932 | 2.5*** | 34.3 | 33.7*** |
| **Birth order** | | | | | |
| 1® | 1713 | 0 | 0 | 28.5 | 29.8 |
| 2 | 944 | −0.451 | 0.64*** | 22.4 | 21.3*** |
| 3+ | 492 | −1.166 | 0.3*** | 12 | 11.7*** |

| Background characteristics | No. of women | B | Odds ratio | Unadjusted probabilities (in percent) | Predicted probabilities (in percent) |
|---|---|---|---|---|---|
| *Socioeconomic factors* | | | | | |
| **Education** | | | | | |
| No schooling® | 655 | 0 | 0 | 12.6 | 19.8 |
| Up to 5 years | 716 | 0.1659 | 1.172 | 15.9 | 22.4 |
| 6–10 years | 1392 | 0.251 | 1.2985 | 25.4 | 24.1 |
| 11+ years | 386 | 0.6437 | 1.9** | 54 | 31.8** |
| **Income (Wealth index)** | | | | | |
| Poor® | 557 | 0 | 0 | 13.2 | 23.7 |
| Middle | 1196 | −0.133 | 0.882 | 15.7 | 21.5 |
| Rich | 1396 | 0.091 | 1.1095 | 35.6 | 25.4 |
| **Religion group** | | | | | |
| Muslims® | 652 | 0 | 0 | 20.9 | 25.9 |
| Hindus | 2463 | −0.154 | 0.8657 | 24.9 | 23.1 |
| Others | 34 | −0.373 | 0.6989 | 23.5 | 19.4 |
| **Social group** | | | | | |
| Scheduled Caste® | 938 | 0 | 0 | 17.6 | 22.8 |
| Scheduled Tribe | 168 | −0.099 | 0.9219 | 14.3 | 21.4 |
| Others | 2043 | 0.0875 | 1.078 | 14.7 | 24.2 |
| **Place of residence** | | | | | |
| Rural® | 2360 | 0 | 0 | 8.7 | 22.6 |
| Urban | 789 | 0.214 | 1.2439 | 29.7 | 26.6 |
| ***Insurance coverage*** | | | | | |
| No® | 3003 | 0 | 0 | 23.1 | 23.6 |
| Yes | 146 | −0.053 | 0.9549 | 45.9 | 22.7 |

*Note: The analysis is based on institutional delivery, (no. of unweighted cases = 3149).*
*The actual probability of C-section delivery in health facilities is about 24% (24.1%, weighted); Cox & Snell R Square = 0.178, Nagelkerke R Square = 0.266; ® Reference category.*
**Significant level at 0.05*
***Significant level at 0.01*
****Significant level at 0.001*
*Sources: Computed from DLHS-3 data files.*

**Table 2.**
*Predicted (adjusted) probabilities of C-section delivery in West Bengal, computed from logistic regression, DLHS-3, 2007–2008, India.*

C-section in private health facilities was 49.6%; that was almost three times higher than public health facilities (18.3%). The place of ANC services did not seem to have a very clear effect on C-section delivery, but the frequency of antenatal visits had a mild effect on C-section delivery; it was mostly found at higher number of ANC visits. The probability of C-section delivery for the older women was higher than younger women after controlling for other variables. With the increase in maternal age, the chances of having C-section delivery also increased. The birth order also was one of the strongest predictors of C-section delivery. With the increase in birth order, the probability of having C-section decreased, which was in the opposite direction to the maternal age. The effect of education was observed, which was mostly found at the higher level of education. A small variation in the probability of C-section delivery was observed between the rural and urban residences, but it was an insignificant factor after controlling for others. The effect of level of income on C-section delivery was mild, so were the effects of religion and caste. Besides, the insurance coverage did not show any significant effect on C-section delivery in this analysis, although it had a large gross effect on C-section delivery in bivariate analysis.

## 4. Discussion

This study showed that the actual probability of C-section delivery was about 12% among all deliveries and 24% among all institutional deliveries in West Bengal. The results of logistic regression revealed that the place of delivery, the number of ANC visits, maternal age, birth order and the level of maternal education were the significant factors associated with the C-section delivery. Delivery in private health facilities was the strongest predictor of C-section delivery as expected. This finding is consistent with the findings of previous studies [14, 17, 20, 28, 29, 36, 37]. This finding could be explained in various ways. Firstly, the proprietors of private health facilities are revenue oriented, and they always try to encourage doctors to perform C-section delivery instead of normal delivery because it brings more revenue; secondly, many doctors are also financially motivated and, therefore, advise patients to have C-section; thirdly, generally doctors are very busy persons, engaged in multiple tasks, and, thus, often they perform C-section even before the arrival of the delivery's labour pain, so as to avoid patient call; and fourthly, both doctors and proprietors of private health facilities do not take risks regarding delivery, so doctors perform C-section before the arrival of the actual delivery's labour pain for avoiding any risks. The higher maternal age was also another important significant factor of C-section delivery. This finding is found to be significant in almost all the previous studies [18, 26, 31, 38, 39]. The higher age of women is much more associated with the prolonged labour, unable to progress at the time of birth and foetal distress which could lead to C-section delivery. Birth order (parity) was also another significant factor of C-section delivery. This finding is similar to a large number of studies [15, 27, 40–43]. The pregnancy and delivery complications are higher among the primiparous women or women of lower birth order than women of higher birth order which leads to higher chances of C-section delivery. On the other hand, maternal age and birth order are highly correlated with each other. The probability of having C-section of lower birth order is higher, but once the birth order is controlled, then higher age has greater chances of C-section delivery. So, women of higher age with the low birth order have higher chances to have C-section delivery. Another most important factor of C-section delivery was the level of woman's education. This finding is also consistent with a large number of previous studies [25, 32, 34, 42, 44, 45]. In general, highly educated women are more aware of maternal and child health and quality of care which would lead women to prefer to go to private health facilities for delivering and ultimately lead to have C-section delivery. The higher number of antenatal visits was the significant factor of C-section delivery as expected though the effect was mild. This finding is also consistent with other studies [22, 26, 29, 30, 46]. The higher number of ANC visits might be the result of pregnancy complications which indicates the surgical operation to deliver a baby. The place of residence was not a significant factor in this study. A similar finding has been observed in the study of Kerala, India [31], and in Jordon [47]. These studies argue that well connectivity and availability of health facilities across the state might be the possible reasons for this finding. The level of income, religion, caste systems and insurance coverage did not show a significant effect on C-section delivery.

## 5. Conclusions

From the above analysis, the present study revealed that women's demographic, socioeconomic background characteristics, antenatal care service and delivery care can have an effect on C-section delivery. From the findings of the present study, it could be recommended that there are some steps which may help to reduce or stop the medically unnecessary C-section delivery for the betterment of women and child health and appropriate use of resources. First, it is found that the rates of C-section delivery were almost three times higher in private health sectors than the public health sectors. Therefore, universal guidelines, protocols and medical audit on C-section should be implemented. Further, the public health system should take steps to monitor the reasons of C-section delivery. The results revealed that women at higher age were at more risk for C-section delivery. The results also found that higher educated women were more tend to have C-section delivery. Thus, the maternal and child health-related educational programme should be implemented for educated women as well as uneducated women. Finally, the community health workers should be trained to circulate the awareness about risks and benefits of C-section delivery, so that medically unnecessary C-section deliveries are not requested or demanded by women and their families. One major limitation of this study is that, in the data source (DLHS, 2007–2008), there is no information on whether the C-section delivery was medically indicated or not. Thus, further studies are needed to examine the factors for medically indicated C-section delivery and medically unindicated C-section delivery separately.

## Acknowledgements

We are very grateful to Prof. P.M. Kulkarni for his overall supervision and the Centre for the Study of Regional Development, Jawaharlal Nehru University, for providing the facility to access various journals.

## Conflict of interest

The authors have no conflicts of interest to declare.

## Funding statement

No funding was obtained for this paper.

## Ethical statement

No ethical approval was needed for this paper.
Consent for publication.
Not applicable.

## Availability of data and materials

This study is based on secondary data which was available in public domain.

## Abbreviations

| | |
|---|---|
| ANC | antenatal care |
| CS | caesarean section/C-section |
| DLHS | District Level Household and Facility Survey |
| IIPS | International Institute for Population Sciences |
| WHO | World Health Organization |

## Author details

Rayhan SK* and Somdutta Barua
Centre for the Study of Regional Development, School of Social Sciences, Jawaharlal Nehru University, New Delhi, India

*Address all correspondence to: rayhangog@gmail.com

## References

[1] Belizan JM, Althabe F, Cafferatat ML. Health consequences of the increasing caesarean section rates. Epidemiology. 2007;**18**:485-486

[2] Betrán AP, Merialdi M, Lauer JA, Bing-shun W, Thomas J, Look PV, et al. Rates of caesarean section: Analysis of global, regional and national estimates. Paediatric and Perinatal Epidemiology. 2007;**21**:98-113

[3] Shah A, Fawole B, M'Imunya JM, Amokrane F, Nafiou I, Wolomby J, et al. Cesarean delivery outcomes 97 from the WHO global survey on maternal and perinatal health in Africa. International Journal of Gynecology and Obstetrics. 2009;**107**(3):191-197

[4] Villar J, Carroli G, Zavaleta N, Donner A, Wojdyla D, Faundes A, et al. Maternal and neonatal individual risks and benefits associated with caesarean delivery: Multicentre prospective study. British Medical Journal. 2007;**335**:1025-1029

[5] Hemminki E. Long term maternal health effects of caesarean section. Journal of Epidemiology and Community Health. 1997;**45**:24-28

[6] Perez-Escamilla R, Maulen-Radovan I, Dewey KG. The association between cesarean delivery and breast-feeding outcomes among Mexican women. American Journal of Public Health. 1996;**86**(6):832-836

[7] Lobel M, DeLuca RS. Psychosocial sequelae of caesarean delivery: Review and analysis of their causes and implications. Social Science and Medicine. 2007;**64**:2272-2284

[8] Shearer EL. Cesarean section: Medical benefits and costs. Social Science and Medicine. 1993;**37**(10):1223-1231

[9] WHO. Appropriate technology for birth. Lancet. 1985;**2**:436-437

[10] WHO. WHO Statement on Caesarean Section Rates. 2014. pp. 1-8. Available from: www.Who.Int/Reproductivehealth/

[11] International Institute for Population Sciences (IIPS). District Level Household and Facility Survey (DLHS-3), 2007-08. Mumbai, India: IIPS; 2010

[12] International Institute for Population Science (IIPS) and Macro International. District Level Household and Facility Survey (DLHS-2), 2002-04. Mumbai, India: IIPS; 2007

[13] International Institute for Population Sciences (IIPS). District Level Household and Facility Survey (DLHS-4), 2012-13, Factsheets. Mumbai, India: IIPS; 2014

[14] Leone T, Padmadas SS, Matthews Z. Community factors affecting rising caesarean section rates in developing countries: An analysis of six countries. Social Science and Medicine. 2008;**67**: 1236-1246

[15] Chacham AS, Perpetuo IHO. The incidence of caesarean deliveries in Belo Horizonte, Brazil: Social and economic determinants. Reproductive Health Matters. 1998;**6**:115-121

[16] Henke RM, Wier LM, Marder WD, Friedman BS, Wong HS. Geographic variation in cesarean delivery in the United States by payer. BMC Pregnancy and Childbirth. 2014;**14**:387

[17] Hopkins K, Amaral E. The role of nonclinical factors in cesarean section rates in Brazil. In: Conference Population Association of America, Philadelphia, UAS; 2005. Available from: http://paa2005.princeton.edu/papers/50741

[18] Stewart-Hall K. An analysis of risk factors associated with high rates

of cesarean births in three selected Northeast Tennessee hospitals (Unpublished master's thesis). Tennessee, USA: East Tennessee State University; 2000

[19] Huang K, Tao F, Faragher B, Raven J, Tolhurst R, Tang S, et al. A mixed-method study of factors associated with differences in caesarean section rates at community level: The case of rural China. Midwifery. 2013;**29**:911-920

[20] Kassak KM, Mohammad AA, Abdallah AM. Opting for a caesarean: What determines the decision? Public Administration and Management. 2009;**13**:100-122

[21] Tebeu PM, Mboudou E, Halle G, Kongnyuy E, Nkwabong E, Fomulu JN. Risk factors of delivery by caesarean section in Cameroon (2003-2004): A regional hospital report. ISRN Obstetrics and Gynecology. 2011;**2011**:1-5

[22] Lee SI, Khang YH, Yun S, Jo MW. Rising rates, changing relationships: Caesarean section and its correlates in South Korea, 1988-2000. BJOG. 2005;**112**:810-812

[23] Parazzini F, Pirotta N, La Vecchia C, Fedele L. Determinants of caesarean section rates in Italy. British Journal of Obstetrics and Gynecology. 1992;**99**:203-206

[24] Kambale Mastaki J. Social predictors of caesarean section births in Italy. African Health Sciences. 2012;**11**:560-565

[25] Prakash KC, Neupane S. Cesarean deliveries among Nepalese mothers: Changes over time 2001-2011 and determinants. Archives of Gynecology and Obstetrics. 2014;**289**(2):421-427

[26] Khawaja M, Kabakian-Khasholian T, Jurdi R. Determinants of caesarean section in Egypt: Evidence from the demographic and health survey. Health Policy. 2004;**69**(3):273-281

[27] Yassin K, Saida G. Levels and determinants of caesarean deliveries in Egypt: Pathways to rationalization. The Internet Journal of World Health and Societal Politics. 2012;7(2):1-13

[28] Gebremedhin S. Trend and socio-demographic differentials of Caesarean section rate in Addis Ababa, Ethiopia: Analysis based on Ethiopia demographic and health surveys data. Reproductive Health. 2014;**11**:14

[29] Mishra US, Ramanathan M. Delivery-related complications and determinants of caesarean section rates in India. Health Policy and Planning. 2002;**17**:90-98

[30] Neuman M, Alcock G, Azad K, Kuddus A, Osrin D, More NS, et al. Prevalence and determinants of caesarean section in private and public health facilities in underserved South Asian communities: Cross-sectional analysis of data from Bangladesh, India and Nepal. BMJ. 2014;**4**(12):e005982

[31] Padmadas SS, Kumar S, Nair SB, Kumari A. Caesarean section delivery in Kerala, India: Evidence from a National Family Health Survey. Social Science and Medicine. 2000;**51**:511-521

[32] Klemetti R, Che X, Gao Y, Raven J, Wu Z, Tang S, et al. Cesarean section delivery among primiparous women in rural China: An emerging epidemic. American Journal of Obstetrics and Gynecology. 2010;**202**:65

[33] Gama SGND, Viellas EF, Schilithz AOC, Filha MMT, Carvalho MLD, Gomes KRO, et al. Factors associated with caesarean section among primiparous adolescents in Brazil, 2011-2012. Cadernos de Saúde Pública. 2014;**30**:S1-S11

[34] Tang S, Li X, Wu Z. Rising caesarean delivery rate in primiparous women in urban China: Evidence from three nationwide household health surveys. The American Journal of Obstetrics and Gynecology. 2006;**195**:1527-1532

[35] Retherford RD, Choe MK. Statistical Model for Causal Analysis. New York, INC: John Wiley and Sons; 1993

[36] Guihard P, Blondel B. Trends in risk factors for caesarean sections in France between 1981 and 1995: Lessons for reducing the rates in the future. British Journal of Obstetrics and Gynaecology. 2001;**108**:48-55

[37] Mossialos E, Allin S, Karras K, Davaki K. An investigation of caesarean sections in three Greek hospitals. The impact of financial incentives and convenience. European Journal of Public Health. 2005;**15**:288-295

[38] Abdul-Rahim HF, Abu-Rmeileh NME, Wick L. Cesarean section deliveries in the occupied Palestinian territory (oPt): An analysis of the 2006 Palestinian Family Health Survey. Health Policy. 2009;**93**:151-156

[39] Räisänen S, Gissler M, Kramer MR, Heinonen S. Influence of delivery characteristics and socioeconomic status on giving birth by caesarean section—A cross sectional study during 2000-2010 in Finland. BMC Pregnancy and Childbirth. 2014;**14**:120

[40] Gomes UA, Silva AA, Bettiol H, Barbieri MA. Risk factors for the increasing caesarean section rate in Southeast Brazil: A comparison of two birth cohorts, 1978-1979 and 1994. International Journal of Epidemiology. 1999;**28**:687-694

[41] Heredia-Pi I, Servan-Mori EE, Wirtz VJ, Avila-Burgos L, Lozano R. Obstetric care and method of delivery in Mexico: Results from the 2012 National Health and Nutrition Survey. PLoS One. 2014;**9**(8):e104166

[42] Patel RR, Peters TJ, Murphy DJ. Prenatal risk factors for caesarean section. Analyses of the ALSPAC cohort of 12 944 women in England. International Journal of Epidemiology. 2005;**34**:353-367

[43] Rahman M, Ahmad Shariff A, Shafie A, Saaid R, Md Tahir R. Determinants of caesarean risk factor in Northern Region of Bangladesh: A multivariate analysis. Iranian Journal of Public Health. 2014;**43**:16-27

[44] Giani U, Bruzzese D, Pugliese A, Saporito M, Triassi M. Risk factors analysis for elective caesarean section in Campania region, Italy. Epidemiologia e Prevenzione. 2011;**35**(2):101-110

[45] Mostafa Kamal SM. Preference for institutional delivery and caesarean sections in Bangladesh. Journal of Health, Population and Nutrition. 2013;**31**:96-109

[46] Koc I. Increased cesarean section rates in Turkey. The European Journal of Contraception and Reproductive Health Care. 2003;**8**:1-10

[47] Khawaja M, Al-Nsour M. Trends in the prevalence and determinants of caesarean section delivery in Jordan: Evidence from three demographic and health surveys, 1990-2002. World Health and Population. 2007;**9**(4):17-28

Chapter 5

# Safe Childbirth and Motherhood in African Great Lakes Region: External Pelvimetry in Nulliparae and Scheduled Caesarean Section

*Jean-Baptiste Kakoma, Xavier Kinenkinda, Fanny Malonga, Joseph Nsambi, Micrette Ngalula, Jeanne Ngoy and Jean Kalibushi*

## Abstract

The authors have carried out a literature review of targeted relevant research with a focus on two countries of the African Great Lakes Region, i.e. Rwanda and the Democratic Republic of the Congo (DRC). The aim was to find a common thread between nulliparity and timely caesarean section through external clinical pelvimetry. Higher rates of nulliparity and caesarean section were found with poor outcome in terms of foeto-maternal prognosis. External clinical pelvimetry presented in Rwandan and Congolese nulliparae the same characteristics during pregnancy and at delivery: lower average values in comparison with multiparae who never experienced caesarean section; average values significantly lower in women who underwent caesarean than in those who delivered naturally; and a gradual and significant decrease in caesarean section rate as pelvic sizes increased. Cephalopelvic disproportion, the main cause of mechanical dystocia, was associated with significantly lower pelvic average values. On the basis of an appropriate tool to predict cephalopelvic disproportion and taking as an illustration of complication the case of obstetrical fistulas, the authors finally advocate the use of the pelvimeter to screen in time pelvises at higher risk for cephalopelvic disproportion in resource-constrained environment.

**Keywords:** childbirth, nulliparae, external pelvimetry, caesarean, African Great Lakes Region

## 1. Introduction

Childbirth is a challenging process that can end in complications that could lead to death, especially when major risk factors are not recognised or dealt with at the right time. It is estimated that about 830 women die every day in the world as a result of complications related to pregnancy or childbirth, and the total number of deceased women in 2015 was estimated at 303,000, although the global maternal mortality ratio decreased by 2.3% per year between 1990 and 2015 [1, 2]. The situation is even worse when it comes to pregnant women in developing countries where deliveries are not most of times attended by skilled health professionals with obvious poor-rich inequalities [3]. Cross-sectional surveys in 80 low and middle-income countries have shown inequalities in the coverage of place of delivery and skilled birth attendance (SBA): SBA deliveries at home and facility non-SBA deliveries were more common in rural than in urban areas and among the poorest in all concerned regions including Sub-Saharan Africa [4]. Another multi-country study showed that only 17.7% of the poorest women versus 54.1% of the richest women used public facilities in Sub-Saharan Africa; and among home births in the poorest, 56% were unattended whereas 41% were attended by a traditional birth attendant [5]. Similar findings have also been reported by other studies [6–9], and in remote areas of limited-resources environment, home-birth practices alone or with the assistance of traditional matrons are the rule [10]. These practices are transmitted from generation to generation in the villages of some developing countries. Globally, about 60 million women give birth every year outside health facilities, primarily at home, and 52 million are not attended by qualified health professionals [11]. The lack of universal skilled attendance leading to lowest emergency obstetric care is explained by a number of reasons, namely the health system deficiency, financial and geographical barriers, mother's educational level, husband's occupation, wrong perception of the household decision maker, hostile behaviour of health personnel, traditional beliefs, and age at first pregnancy [5–8, 12, 13]. Among all pregnant women, nulliparae are at higher risk in abovementioned conditions as unplanned caesarean deliveries leading to adverse foeto-maternal outcomes are not an exception in a poor environment [14, 15]. Therefore, most of caesarean sections are emergency ones, as attending matrons always attempt at all costs to deliver vaginally babies regardless of the situation according to certain ethnocultural beliefs. This perception persists even among immigrant women in developed countries [16]. Consequently, in case of cephalopelvic disproportion, unsuccessful attempts to give birth vaginally result in neglected prolonged labour resulting in an emergency caesarian section in appalling conditions, particularly in the presence of transport and financial barriers as is the most common case. This also happens in health centres of urban areas when the health system is completely disorganised. Thus, foeto-maternal morbidity and mortality become higher to the point of making hospitals statistics alarming. In one hand, newborn death, uterine rupture and obstetric fistula are among complications with the saddest impact on a surviving primiparous woman and her family with regard to the pronatalist African culture. In the other hand, cephalopelvic disproportion due to generally contracted pelvis or large foetal head circumference is one of caesarean section indications in nulliparae and pregnant women aged less than 19 [17–20]; and this should also be the case in settings characterised by early marriages and lack of appropriate pregnancy monitoring. Besides, it is also known that external pelvimetry is nowadays controversial and no longer in favour with many obstetricians [21, 22], now that new, more powerful diagnostic tools, e.g. CT pelvimetry using multi detector CT and magnetic resonance-based serial pelvimetry [23, 24], are available and which will take time to reach pregnant women in resource-limited areas. Meanwhile, results from some surveys in Sub-Saharan Africa and elsewhere have shown a significant relationship between some external pelvic diameters and cephalopelvic disproportion or dystocia indication for caesarean section in nulliparae [25–28]. Our aim is in fine to advocate, on the basis of our findings in the African Great Lakes Region, the reintroduction of pelvimeter as a cheap and helpful tool in hands of well-trained health professionals, in order to promote scheduled caesarean sections, and therefore to prevent harmful outcomes such as newborn death, uterine rupture and obstetric fistula in young mothers leaving in resource-limited environment.

## 2. Context

Apart from background data, findings from surveys and studies concerned in next sections have been collected in two countries of the African Great Lakes Region at the heart of Africa; namely, Rwanda and the Democratic Republic of the Congo. Rwanda is a tiny and landlocked country, which is the more densely populated (519/km$^2$) in Sub-Saharan Africa. Its infrastructure and qualified manpower was greatly impacted by the 1994 genocide in general and specifically in the health sector [29]. About 90% of population is presently covered by the national mutual health insurance, while the country was steadily moving towards reaching some MDG by 2015 deadline [30]. Surely, financial dependence on external assistance is still high, and the shortage of human resources for health still challenging. However, Rwanda is one of the rare African countries that have allocated an appreciated part of their national budget to health, and since more than a decade, efforts and innovative solutions are ongoing to train, deploy and retain health professionals, should education programmes and retention strategies be regularly and appropriately readjusted, as far as human resources remain a tremendous challenge in the public sector [31]. On the whole, Rwanda is rather doing well economically and in the social sectors. The Democratic Republic of the Congo (DRC), as far as it is concerned, is one of the "Big Five" countries in Africa with a surface area estimated at 2,345,000 km$^2$ and a population of more than 80 million. DRC was all destined to be one of the best performing countries on the continent given its diversified natural resources, the proportion of actual qualified manpower and its basic infrastructure of departure at the time of its independence (30th June 1960). Apart from few ephemeral peaks of light development, this country, undermined by endless rebellions and the neglect of its political class, ended up being one of the failed countries of the world [32]. Its health system is a total mess: no evident leadership and vision, and very far from a minimum of transparency and accountability. As a result, we are witnessing a resurgence of old epidemics, the activation of old endemics, the spread of sexual violence and the worsening of the Ebola virus infection. We are not far from a "not assistance to a people in danger" situation!

## 3. Childbirth, motherhood and nulliparity

### 3.1 Background

There are many risk factors that can compromise childbirth and motherhood as far as emergency caesarean section is concerned in limited resources settings. Among these is parity, namely nulliparity and multiparity [33, 34]. Concerning nulliparity in general, it is worldwide known that nulliparous women are at higher risk of pregnancy, delivery and neonatal complications. They are prone to anaemia, pre-eclampsia, anal sphincter injury, operative vaginal delivery, postcaeserean surgical site infection, dystocia, caesarean delivery, inadequate uterine contractions, foetal malposition, cephalopelvic disproportion, premature labour, low birth weight, funisitis, neonatal morbidity, perinatal mortality, induction of labour, routine episiotomy, hypertensive complications, and postpartum haemorrhage [33–42]. The situation is similar for teenagers who are pregnant [43]. All these cases become very worrying when it comes to pregnant women living in remote areas of conflict or postconflict regions, and even in urban areas in absence of qualified health professionals, suitable motivation and appropriate equipment. Rwanda is a postconflict region while DRC is still a conflict region, especially the eastern part of the country. The situation is most crucial in DRC when Rwanda is doing well as far as Universal Health Coverage and MDG achievement are concerned [44, 45].

### 3.2 Findings in Rwanda and DRC

A recent health facility-based cross-sectional study has been carried out in Rwanda (Kigali and Northern Province) from 2014 to 2015 through structured interviews and medical records ($n = 817$). This study has shown a higher rate of nulliparity (41.1%) as assessed through self-reported data from postpartum women [46]. This should not be shocking, as there are many young marriages in Rwanda after the 1994 genocide for reasons that are understandable. However, this high rate of nulliparity is also accompanied by high levels of risk associated with first pregnancy and childbirth. A previous cross-sectional case–control study (n = 600) at Muhima District Hospital in Kigali has shown in 2009 that nulliparous women were at higher risk than multiparae with regard to many obstetrical and neonatal outcomes. Nulliparous women were significantly prone to: lower weight ($p = 0.016$); malaria crisis ($p = 0.031$); induction of labour ($p = 0.008$); caesarean delivery ($p < 0.001$); episiotomy ($p < 0.001$); failure of descent ($p = 0.037$); transfer to neonatal care (0.025), and lower average birth weight ($p < 0.001$) [41].

In DRC, a recent cross-sectional and analytical study of singleton births in postpartum women ($n = 4197$) reported, from December 2013 to May 2014, a nulliparity rate of 19.9% in 10 referral maternity hospitals in Lubumbashi, Upper Katanga Province. Primiparous women (i.e. nulliparous before delivery) as compared with multiparae were during pregnancy at higher risk for: high blood pressure (OR = 1.91 [1.32–2.74]); malpresentation (OR = 1.95 [1.16–3.17]); oxytocin use (OR = 2.03 [1.64–2.52]); caesarean section (OR = 2.04 [1.47–2.83]); episiotomy (OR = 11.89 [8.61–16.43]); eclampsia (OR = 4.21 [1.55–11.44]); lower rate of 5th minute APGAR score (OR = 1.55 [1.03–2.32]); and higher rate of early neonatal mortality (OR = 1.80 [1.08–2.98]) [47].

## 4. Caesarean section delivery

### 4.1 Background

It has been suggested by the World Health Organisation (WHO) that caesarean section rate should range between 5 and 15% in order to benefit to mother, foetus and newborn [48, 49]. Therefore, a rate above 15% is assimilated to unjustified use of surgical delivery, while a rate below 5% reveals a population's lack of access to medical technology [31]; besides, evidence based results show that there is no correlation, at population level, between caesarean rates higher than 10% and reduction of maternal and newborn mortality [50]. Nowadays, more and more claims around the world stigmatise the shocking rising trends of caesarean section, especially in private sectors as 'on demand caesarean section' or 'caesarean section on maternal request' has become a routine indication in medical practice [51, 52]. Given maternal and perinatal complications associated with caesarean section, efforts are recommended to provide surgical delivery to only women in real need, assuming that the medical environment is appropriate [50]. Thus, there is a need to be more cautious as regards caesarean section indications and quantity regulation in order to reduce health costs as well as maternal and foetal risks [50, 51]. In this regard, the prevailing situation in the countries of African Great Lakes region is generally frightening, particularly in DRC given the conflict or postconflict environment.

### 4.2 Findings in Rwanda and DRC

For more than a decade, different scientific reports in Rwanda have revealed higher rates of caesarean compared to the upper limit (15%) for caesarean section set by WHO. In 2006 and 2007, two descriptive cross-sectional studies found caesarean section rates of 41% and 33.7% in a urban national reference hospital (Kigali city) and a rural district hospital (Northern Province), respectively [53, 54]. Two other cross-sectional studies (descriptive and case-control) conducted in 2008 and 2009 have also shown higher rates of caesarean, i.e. 21.05% and 28% (versus 10.7% in multiparae), in nulliparous women from a rural area (Huye/Southern Province; n = 152) and Kigali city (n = 600), respectively [41, 55]. In DRC, a retrospective study was carried out in Lubumbashi on 34,199 deliveries from five referral hospitals for a period of five years (2009 to 2013). This study noticed an overall caesarean section rate of 10.65% with a slight increase from 2009 (10.24%) to 2013 (11.38%). Almost one caesarean section out of two (48.6%) occurred in an emergency context and the majority (51.4%) of caesareans after unsuccessful attempt to give birth naturally. Unfortunately, the 11% increase in caesareans did not bring any benefit in terms of foeto-maternal prognosis as there was no significant change in perinatal mortality rate whereas overall maternal mortality rate jumped from 2.3‰ in 2009 to 6.4‰ in 2013, which was a highly significant 317.5% increase (p = 0.005) [56]. Five months later (December 2013–May 2014), an abovementioned analytical cross-sectional study on primiparae (nulliparae before delivery) reported in the same environment a caesarean rate of 13.03% (versus 6.84% in multiparae) in postpartum primiparous women with a poor neonatal outcome [47].

## 5. External pelvimetry and ways of delivery in nulliparae and multiparae

### 5.1 Background

Since more than two centuries, women pelvic architecture and pelvic girdle measurements have been a matter of scientific concern for obstetricians. Women pelvis and pelvimetry have been deeply studied in the eighteenth and the nineteenth century by a number of eminent scientists among whom Hendrik Van Deventer, Jean Louis Baudelocque, Gustav Adolf Michaelis, Franz Karl Joseph Naegele, Stein Jr., and Carl Conrad Theodor Litzman [57]. Different types of pelvimeters became common tools in maternity wards and delivery rooms. In the past, young trainees in medicine, assistants in obstetrics and midwives constantly and regularly used these pelvimeters, which were familiar to them. Gradually, this instrument disappeared from hospital maternities to end up only in a few health centres held by old nuns. This was the case in Rwanda and DRC. Moreover, the effectiveness of pelvimeter has for some time become questionable for most obstetricians under the pressure of advances in technology during the ending twentieth century and given the alleged lack of satisfactory scientific evidence [21, 22]. However, we are still living in a world where health care equity and access to quality health care remain to date an unattainable dream worldwide and even when it comes to different social classes within some industrialised countries. Therefore, it is the duty of scientists and men in the field to look for simple ways and inexpensive tools to help the many left behind, especially young pregnant women in resource-constrained countries in an environment dominated by all kinds of barriers. It is in this context that a number of studies have been conducted on the relationship between anthropometric parameters including height, weight as well as external pelvic diameters and ways of delivery in some parts of the world, and more particularly in Sub-Saharan Africa, Central Africa and African Great Lakes region [25–28]. Reported findings below are products of researches conducted in Rwanda (Southern Province and Kigali city) and DRC (Lubumbashi, Upper Katanga Province).

## 5.2 Findings in Rwanda and DRC

Results from Rwanda and DRC were obtained from research projects carried out either within the framework of an institutional cooperation (Southern Province of Rwanda) or as requirements for academic degrees of master's or PhD in medicine (Kigali/Rwanda and Lubumbashi/DRC) under the scrutiny of a same supervisor in 2007, 2010 and 2017. Data were collected at antenatal care clinics and at admission to delivery rooms in nulliparae and multiparae. Statistics central values and spread were identified for different external pelvic diameters and two other anthropometric parameters (height and weight). Concerned pelvic parameters were: intercrestal or biiliac diameter, interspinous diameter, intertrochanteric diameter, anteroposterior (Baudelocque's) diameter or external conjugate, intertuberous or bi-ischiatic diameter, and the base of Trillat's triangle or prepubic diameter. Only multiparae with no previous caesarean experience and nulliparae without pelvic malformations were selected so that measurements in multiparae were considered as base normal sizes while those in nulliparae could be considered as a mixture of normal and abnormal pelvic sizes as long as they had not yet faced the process of childbirth in the same environment (rural and urban areas in Rwanda, and urban area in DRC). Later on, delivery ways were observed in only nulliparous women with a single foetus in vertex presentation.

### *5.2.1 Pelvic measurements in multiparae and nulliparae in the Southern Province of Rwanda*

Huye District in the Southern Province of Rwanda served as the framework of a cross-sectional and analytical study in nulliparae ($n$ = 312) and multiparae ($n$ = 314) at prenatal care settings on randomly fixed days from December 2007 to January 2008. Pelvic measurements were taken and average pelvic sizes in multiparae who have always delivered per vaginam were compared to those in nulliparae (Student's $t$ test). The aim of the study was to describe and characterise external pelvic parameters in Rwandan pregnant women in a rural area. Average sizes were significantly greater in multiparae than in nulliparae except for the intertrochanter diameter and the base of the Trillat's triangle (**Table 1**). These preliminary findings suggested the fact that external pelvic diameters of multiparous women without previous caesarean experience would belong to pelvises best suited for delivery. It is worth noting that measurements in both multiparae and nulliparae were normally distributed (Kolmogorov-Smirnov test) [58].

| Diameters (cm) | Multiparae ($N$ = 314) Mean ± SD | Nulliparae ($N$ = 312) Mean ± SD | $p^*$ |
|---|---|---|---|
| Intercrestal (biiliac) | 23.92 ± 1.56 | 23.38 ± 1.60 | 0.001 |
| Interspinous | 22.20 ± 1.60 | 21.74 ± 1.58 | 0.001 |
| Intertrochanteric | 27.32 ± 1.98 | 27.04 ± 2.12 | 0.087 |
| Intertuberous | 9.67 ± 0.68 | 9.22 ± 0.76 | 0.001 |
| Anteroposterior | 17.92 ± 1.61 | 17.48 ± 1.50 | 0.001 |
| Base of Trillat's triangle | 13.43 ± 0.84 | 13.78 ± 1.00 | 0.001 |

**Student's t test.*

**Table 1.**
*Comparison of pelvic diameters between Rwandan multiparae and nulliparae in the Southern Province.*

### *5.2.2 Pelvic measurements in multiparae and nulliparae in Kigali City/Rwanda*

A cross-sectional and analytical study was also carried out in Kigali City (Kigali University Teaching Hospital and Muhima District Hospital) from May 2009 to June 2010 in nulliparae ($n$ = 318) and multiparae ($n$ = 303) at admission in delivery rooms. One of the specific objectives of the study was also to describe and characterise pelvic and anthropometric parameters in Rwandan pregnant women in an urban area. Student's t test was used to compare average values observed in multiparae and nulliparae. Average sizes in multiparae who never experienced caesarean section were also significantly greater than in nulliparae for all considered pelvic diameters (**Table 2**). The same abovementioned implication about pelvis suitability in multiparae was suggested while average pelvic sizes in both multiparae and nulliparae were smaller in rural women from the rural area (Southern Province) than in their urban counterparts (Kigali City). Nutritional status was suggested as the factor that would explain this difference [59].

| Diameters (cm) | Multiparae ($N$ = 318) Mean ± SD | Nulliparae ($N$ = 303) Mean ± SD | $p^*$ |
|---|---|---|---|
| Intercrestal | 26.58 ± 0.01 | 24.33 ± 0.16 | 0.327 |
| Interspinous | 24.04 ± 0.09 | 23.73 ± 0.17 | 0.014 |
| Intertrochanteric | 29.09 ± 0.13 | 28.88 ± 0.20 | <0.001 |
| Intertuberous | 12.90 ± 0.10 | 12.25 ± 0.13 | <0.001 |
| Anteroposterior | 18.62 ± 0.18 | 18.14 ± 0.12 | <0.001 |
| Base of Trillat's triangle | 15.27 ± 0.10 | 14.39 ± 0.13 | <0.001 |

**Student's t test.*

**Table 2.**
*Comparison of pelvic diameters between Rwandan multiparae and nulliparae in Kigali city.*

### *5.2.3 Pelvic measurements in multiparae and nulliparae in DRC*

A descriptive cross-sectional study as part of a large research project in the city of Lubumbashi was carried out from February 2016 to August 2017 in nulliparae ($n$ = 535) and multiparae ($n$ = 938) on pelvic and anthropometric parameters. Data were collected at antenatal clinics and admission to delivery rooms in seven maternities. The aim of the study was among others to profile external pelvic sizes in nulliparae and multiparae who used to give birth naturally. At first glance, external pelvic diameters sizes showed also a greater or lesser difference between Congolese multiparae and nulliparae in Lubumbashi (**Table 3**). The same deduction made about pelvis suitability for Rwandan women could also be applied to Congolese women [60].

| Pelvic measurements (cm) | Multiparae ($N$ = 938) Mean ± SD | Nulliparae ($N$ = 535) Mean ± SD |
|---|---|---|
| Intercrestal | 26.02 ± 2. 17 | 24.69 ± 2.28 |
| Interspinous | 22.94 ± 2. 37 | 21. 79 ± 3.78 |
| Intertrochanteric | 29.81 ± 2.72 | 29.26 ± 2.98 |
| Intertuberous | 10.22 ± 0.94 | 9.77 ± 1.51 |
| Anteroposterior | 20.22 ± 1.32 | 19.94 ± 1.92 |
| Base of Trillat's triangle | 13.04 ± 1,31 | 13.00 ± 1.82 |

**Table 3.**
*Pelvic measurements in multiparae and nulliparae in DRC.*

### 5.2.4 External pelvic diameters in nulliparae and caesarean section in Rwanda

A prospective, longitudinal and descriptive study was conducted in 152 Rwandan parturients out of the 312 nulliparae who participated in a previous study on external clinical pelvimetry at antenatal care settings in Huye District/Southern Province of the country [58]. From December 2007 to April 2008, the investigators went over all the health centres and hospitals in the Huye District to look for deliveries of nulliparae involved in the abovementioned survey. Apart from pelvic and anthropometric measurements (already taken at antenatal care settings), the only considered medical parameters were the mode of delivery, the vertex presentation of the foetus, and singleton live birth. Deliveries and caesarean sections were blindly performed by midwives, general practitioners and specialists who did not take part in the survey. Yates' chi-square test was used to compare observed proportions. Results showed that caesarean section rates were more or less higher for values below the predefined thresholds for pelvic diameter sizes, i.e. average minus one standard deviation (**Table 4**). The difference was only significant for the base of the Trillat's triangle and the intertuberous diameter [61].

| Diameters (cm) | | Way of delivery | | $p^*$ |
|---|---|---|---|---|
| | | Per vaginam ($N$ = 120) | Caesarean ($N$ = 32) | |
| Intercrestal | <22 | 11 (68.7%) | 5 (31.3%) | 0.290 |
| | ≥22 | 100 (80.1%) | 27 (19.9%) | |
| Interspinous | <20 | 7 (77.8%) | 2 (22.2%) | 0.929 |
| | ≥20 | 113 (79%) | 30 (21%) | |
| Intertrochanteric | <28 | 23 (71.9%) | 9 (28.1%) | 0.269 |
| | ≥28 | 97 (80.8%) | 23 (19.2%) | |
| Intertuberous | <8 | 4 (44.4%) | 5 (55.6%) | 0.009 |
| | ≥ 8 | 116 (81.1%) | 27 (18.9%) | |
| Anteroposterior | <17 | 23 (71.9%) | 9 (28.1%) | 0.260 |
| | ≥17 | 97 (80.83%) | 23 (19.17%) | |
| Base of Trillat's triangle | <11 | 0 (0.00%) | 4 (100%) | 0.001 |
| | ≥11 | 120 (81.1%) | 28 (18.9%) | |

*$\chi^2$ test with Yates' correction.*

**Table 4.**
*Pelvic diameters and caesarean section in Rwandan nulliparae.*

### 5.2.5 External pelvic diameters in nulliparae and caesarean section in DRC

A descriptive cross-sectional study was conducted in Lubumbashi from February 2016 to August 2017 in 400 nulliparae in order to compare ways of delivery associated with different sizes of two external pelvic diameters, namely the intertuberous diameter and the base of the Trillat's triangle. Pelvic measurements were already taken at antenatal care settings and the following parameters were collected after delivery: the mode of delivery, the vertex presentation of the foetus, and singleton live birth. Deliveries and caesarean sections were blindly performed by midwives, general practitioners and specialists who did not take part in the survey. Yates' chi-square and Student's $t$ test were used to compare observed proportions and average values, respectively. Lowest dimensions of the base of the Trillat's triangle or prepubic diameter (i.e. <11 cm) and of the intertuberous diameter (i.e. <8 cm) were associated with higher caesarean section rates (i.e. 69.23 and 91.67% respectively) while highest dimensions (i.e. ≥16 and ≥12 cm respectively) were associated with lower caesarean section rates (8.33 and 5% respectively) in nulliparae, and the difference was highly significant. On the whole, there was a gradual decrease in caesarean section rates as the size of the base of Trillat's triangle and of the intertuberous diameter increased (**Tables 5** and **6**). Related average diameter sizes were also significantly lower in women who delivered by caesarean section, i.e. 11.99 ± 1.37 cm versus 12.82 ± 1.39 cm for the prepubic diameter, and 9.10 ± 1.23 cm versus 10.27 ± 1.10 cm for the intertuberous diameter ($p < 0.001$) [62].

At the same time and under the same conditions, 453 nulliparae were involved in a concomitant descriptive cross-sectional study about other external pelvic diameters. The same relationship was reproduced with regard to average sizes of pelvic diameters, which were significantly lower in women who have undergone caesarean than in those who gave birth naturally (**Table 7**) [63].

| Trillat's triangle base (cm) | Caesarean | | Vaginal delivery | | Total | | $p^*$ |
|---|---|---|---|---|---|---|---|
| | *N* | % | *N* | % | *N* | % | |
| <11 | 18 | 69.23 | 8 | 30.77 | 26 | 100 | <0.001 |
| 11–11.9 | 28 | 38.89 | 44 | 61.11 | 72 | 100 | |
| 12–12.9 | 26 | 24.30 | 81 | 75.70 | 107 | 100 | |
| 13–13.9 | 19 | 19.39 | 79 | 80.61 | 98 | 100 | |
| 14–14.9 | 10 | 17.54 | 47 | 82.46 | 57 | 100 | |
| 15–15.9 | 3 | 10.71 | 25 | 89.29 | 28 | 100 | |
| ≥16 | 1 | 8.33 | 11 | 91.67 | 12 | 100 | |

*$^*\chi^2$ test with Yates' correction.*

**Table 5.**
*Trillat's triangle base and obstetrical outcome in nulliparae in DRC.*

| Intertuberous diameter (cm) | Caesarean | | Vaginal delivery | | Total | | $p^*$ |
|---|---|---|---|---|---|---|---|
| | *N* | % | *N* | % | *N* | % | |
| <7.9 | 11 | 91.67 | 1 | 8.33 | 12 | 100 | <0.001 |
| 8–8.9 | 23 | 69.70 | 10 | 30.30 | 33 | 100 | |
| 9–9.9 | 30 | 29.70 | 71 | 70.30 | 101 | 100 | |
| 10–10.9 | 31 | 24.60 | 95 | 75.40 | 126 | 100 | |
| 11–11.9 | 8 | 9.09 | 80 | 90.91 | 88 | 100 | |
| ≥ 12 | 2 | 5.00 | 38 | 95.00 | 40 | 100 | |

*$^*\chi^2$ test with Yates' correction.*

**Table 6.**
*Intertuberous diameter and obstetrical outcome in nulliparae in DRC.*

| Pelvic diameters (cm) | Caesarean Mean ± SD (Median) | Vaginal delivery Mean ± SD (Median) | $p^*$ |
|---|---|---|---|
| Biiliac | 25.46 ± 2.10 (25 cm) | 24.14 ± 1.92 (24 cm) | <0.001 |
| Antero-superior iliac interspinous | 21.80 ± 2 (22 cm) | 23.03 ± 2.31 (23 cm) | <0.001 |
| Intertrochanter | 27.68 ± 2.24 (28 cm) | 29.44 ± 2.82 (29 cm) | <0.001 |
| Baudelocque | 18.34 ± 1.77 (18 cm) | 20.78 ± 1.88 (20 cm) | <0.001 |
| Conjugata vera pelvis# | 9.35 ± 1.76 (9 cm) | 11.79 ± 1.92 (11 cm) | <0.001 |

*#Baudelocque's diameter minus9 cm.*
**Wilcoxon signed-rank test.*

**Table 7.**
*Pelvic diameters and obstetrical outcome in nulliparae in DRC.*

### *5.2.6 Caesarean section indications and external pelvic diameters in Rwanda*

A cross-sectional and analytical study was made on data collected from 32 operated parturients among 152 nulliparae who gave birth with singleton pregnancy at term and vertex presentation within the three first months of the abovementioned prospective longitudinal survey in the Southern Province of Rwanda [61]. Anthropometric measurements (external pelvic diameters in cm) were collected at first antenatal care consultation. At childbirth, midwives and physicians monitored labour in a blind way and the following data were collected after delivery by the investigators: way of delivery (per vaginam or caesarean section), and caesarean section indication. Student's *t* test was used to compare mean values from a normally distributed population (Kolmogorov-Smirnov test). This study showed a relationship between external pelvic sizes and caesarean section indications related to obstructed labour due to pelvic dystocia. Clinically diagnosed pelvis contraction was characterised by smaller average measurements in comparison with other caesarean section indications. Apart from biiliac (intercrestal) diameter, observed differences were statistically significant for all other external pelvic diameters, i.e. antero-superior iliac interspinous, intertrochanter, Baudelocque's, and intertuberous (**Table 8**) [55].

| Diameters (cm) | Contracted pelvis ($N = 9$) | Other indications ($N = 23$) | Mean difference | $p^*$ |
|---|---|---|---|---|
| Biiliac | 22.83 ± 2.59 | 23.45 ± 1.34 | 0.62 | 0.375 |
| Antero-superior Iliac interspinous | 20.87 ± 1.59 | 21.94 ± 1.15 | 1.07 | 0.043 |
| Intertrochanter | 25.70 ± 2.56 | 27.72 ± 2.26 | 2.02 | 0.036 |
| Baudelocque | 16.20 ± 1.17 | 18.50 ± 1.31 | 2.30 | 0.001 |
| Intertuberous | 7.76 ± 0.43 | 9.26 ± 0.68 | 1.50 | 0.001 |
| Trillat's base | 12.17 ± 2.26 | 13.98 ± 0.93 | 1.81 | 0.003 |

**Student's t test.*

**Table 8.**
*External pelvimetry and caesarean section indication in Rwandan nulliparae.*

### *5.2.7 Pelvic dystocia and external pelvic diameters in DRC*

A cross-sectional descriptive study with an analytical component in nulliparae ($n = 535$) was conducted in seven referral hospitals in the city of Lubumbashi from February 2016 to August 2017 in order to describe the morphological characteristics (anthropometric and pelvimetric externally) and to identify their thresholds for the specification of appropriate determinants and the development of a predictive score for the type of delivery (vaginal versus caesarean) in pregnant women. Only 535 nulliparae who gave birth with singleton pregnancy at term and vertex presentation were involved in this study; and only caesarean sections indicated for mechanical dystocia were considered. A predictive score (TABIT score: TA for "taille", i.e. height; BI for "bi-ischiatique", i.e. intertuberous; and T for "Trillat", i.e. prepubic diameter) was defined after logistic modelling to predict the occurrence of mechanical dystocia. Three criteria emerged as predictors (determinants) of mechanical dystocia: maternal height < 150 cm (OR adjusted = 2.96 [1.49–5.87]), bi-ischiatic or intertuberous diameter < 8 cm (OR adjusted = 15.96 [3.46–73.56]) and Trillat's triangle base or prepubic diameter < 11 cm (OR adjusted = 2.34 [1.36–4.01]). The total number of points attributed to the three determinants was 5 (<2 = low risk,

2–3 = moderate risk, and >3 = high risk). This scoring system had a sensitivity of 23. 81%, a specificity of 97.80%, a predictive value of a positive test of 76. 92%, and that of a negative test of 80.65%. The area under the ROC curve was 0.6549, within the range of acceptable values [64]. Although this tool can already be operational in conjunction with clinical data, efforts will be made to improve this scoring system by including one additional parameter to increase sensitivity, and uterine height as a proxy for foetal parameters is the most targeted obstetrical variable. In so doing, we could have a simple and cheap tool, usable by any health professional at antenatal clinics and after parturients admission to delivery room.

## 6. Home-birth practice and vaginal childbirth at all costs

### 6.1 Background

Home-birth practice usually happens in remote rural areas where qualified health professionals are rare, even absent or unknown; this is the case in most conflict areas of DRC and particularly in Upper Katanga province for several years past. In these conditions, the matrons are at work without any restraint. The tacit rule is to give birth whatever the cost by natural way. In a context of financial and geographical barriers, and facing the lack of qualified health staff coupled with the lack of adequate infrastructure and equipment, one has no choice but to wait for a possible favourable evolution of childbirth under the supervision of the matrons or any other person in charge of the parturients in the community who often do not hesitate to resort to the traditional medication. All this may result in obstructed labour or dystocia, which often occurs when the foetal head is stuck in the mother's pelvis, interrupting blood flow to the surrounding tissues. This results afterwards in prolonged ischemia which may progress to tissue necrosis, the fall of which leads to fistulas formation. Most of the time, cephalopelvic disproportion, which is one of the most frequent indications of caesarean section in nulliparae in our environment [41, 55, 56], is the primum movens of this process. Obstetric fistulas (urogenital) have debilitating consequences such as urinary incontinence, faecal incontinence or both, and damage to the vulva and thighs. They bring about well-known social ostracism and dehumanising stigmatisation with a urge impact on social, psychological, and sexual life of patients, more particularly in a context of extreme socioeconomic precariousness. In developed countries the incidence of vesicovaginal fistula is 0.3–2%, while it is not known in developing countries because of the underreporting of cases; and if it can be annually estimated, only a certain portion can benefit from treatment [65–67].

### 6.2 Findings in DRC

A descriptive cross-sectional study was carried out from September 2009 to December 2013 in Upper Katanga Province (DRC) after five mass treatment campaigns in six health districts (Pweto, Kilwa, Mitwaba, Kasenga, Kashobwe and Lubumbashi). This study that involved 242 patients depicted a gloomy situation about sociodemographic and obstetrical characteristics of these patients at the time of fistula: 40.1% aged <20, 90.6% of nulliparae, 94.6% of vaginal delivery; 85.9% of ≥48 hours labour duration, 70.7% of home-birth practice, 93.4% of neonatal mortality, and 71.5% of patients living alone. Clinical parameters related to fistula were as follows: a history of fistula of 5 years and more (33.5%), vesico-vaginal fistula (96%) and failure of fistula repair (14%) [68]. This situation is only the tip of an iceberg as not all women concerned could be reached by the awareness campaigns.

Therefore, it is obvious that obstetric fistula is a real public health problem in the DRC, and particularly in nulliparae. Concerning prolonged labour and caesarean section performed under inappropriate conditions, other equally serious complications are uterine rupture, which compromises the reproductive capacity, as well as the high maternal and perinatal morbidity and mortality. And yet all this would be avoidable if we could act upstream by predicting the outcome of the pregnancy (i.e. the way of delivery) with a high probability so that the maternal and perinatal prognosis could be considerably improved.

## 7. Conclusion

Results from studies on childbirth and motherhood in two countries of the African Great Lakes Region, namely Rwanda and the Democratic Republic of the Congo, highlighted high rates of nulliparity, which have had a deleterious effect on obstetrical and perinatal outcomes. Higher rates of caesarean section have been observed, especially in nulliparous women. One of the most frequent indications of caesarean section was cephalopelvic disproportion that leads to prolonged and obstructed labour in a context of lack of qualified health professionals. As most of the time, cephalopelvic disproportion results from pelvis inadequacy to allow the foetus to negotiate the birth canal, pelvic diameters represent the essential parameters to be taken into account in predicting the route of delivery and preventing serious maternal and perinatal complications following caesarean sections in poor conditions. In Rwanda as well as in DRC a significant relationship has been found between accessible external pelvic diameters and obstetrical outcomes (natural delivery and caesarean section), while cephalopelvic disproportion was the main caesarean section indication. This relies heavily on the question of the usefulness of pelvic evaluation in nulliparae during pregnancy in countries with limited resources, especially in remote areas. It is therefore a noble human duty to seek appropriate, efficient and evidence-based solutions and tools to help improve the health of the mother-child couple, which is part of all global goals. In this context, the early detection of nulliparae at higher risk of cephalopelvic disproportion, as soon as they are pregnant, would protect them and their infants by avoiding unscheduled caesarean sections and complications that could have life-long consequences or could endanger life. We believe that pelvimeter, this simple affordable tool, could be, in expert hands, one of those needed tools in resource-limited settings. Pregnant youngsters could thus benefit from the advantageous effects of a timely caesarean section and enjoy a safe motherhood, and besides, childbirth would not at all be a very dangerous event for both mother and child.

## Author details

Jean-Baptiste Kakoma[1,2,3*], Xavier Kinenkinda[1], Fanny Malonga[1], Joseph Nsambi[1], Micrette Ngalula[1], Jeanne Ngoy[1] and Jean Kalibushi[3]

1 Department of Obstetrics and Gynaecology, University of Lubumbashi School of Medicine, Democratic Republic of the Congo

2 Department of Epidemiology, University of Lubumbashi School of Public Health, Democratic Republic of the Congo

3 Department of Obstetrics and Gynaecology, University of Rwanda College of Medicine and Health Sciences, Rwanda

*Address all correspondence to: jbszkakoma2016@gmail.com

## References


[1] WHO. Maternal mortality Key facts. 16 Feb 2018. Available from: https://www.who.int/news-room/fact-sheets/detail/maternal-mortality [Accessed: 24 August 2019]

[2] Alkema L, Chou D, Hogan D, Zhang S, Moller AB, Gemmill A, et al. Global, regional, and national levels and trends in maternal mortality between 1990 and 2015, with scenario-based projections to 2030: a systematic analysis by the UN Maternal Mortality Estimation Inter-Agency Group. Lancet. 2016;**387**(10017):462-474

[3] Houweling TAJ, Ronsmans C, Campbell OMR, Kunst AE. Huge poor-rich inequalities in maternity care: An international comparative study of maternity and child care in developing countries. Bulletin of the World Health Organization. 2007;**85**:745-754

[4] Joseph G, Da Silva ICM, Wehrmeister FC, Barros AJD, Victora CG. Inequalities in the coverage of place of delivery and skilled birth attendance: analyses of cross-sectional surveys in 80 low and middle-income countries. Reproductive Health. 2016;**13**:77. DOI: 10.1186/s12978-016-0192-2 [Accessed: 23 August 2019]

[5] Montagu D, Yamey G, Visconti A, Harding A, Yoong J. Where do poor Women in developing countries give birth? A multi-country analysis of demographic and health survey data. PLoS One. 2011;**6**(2):e17155. DOI: 10.1371/journal.pone.0017155 [Accessed: 15 October 2019]

[6] Ahmed S, Creanga AA, Gillespie DG, Tsui AO. Economic status, education and empowerment: Implications for maternal health service utilization in developing countries. PLoS One. 2010;**5**(6):e11190. DOI: 10.1371/journal.pone.0011190 [Accessed: 15 October 2019]

[7] Idris SH, Gwarzo UMD, Shehu AU. Determinants of place of delivery among women in a semi-urban settlement in Zaria, Northern Nigeria. Annals of African Medicine. 2006;**5**(2):68-72

[8] Chanza D, Chirwa E, Maluwa A, Malata A, Masache G. Factors affecting the choice for home deliveries in Malawi. African Journal of Midwifery and Women's Health. 23 Sep 2013;**6**(3):125-130. DOI: 10.12968/ajmw.2012.6.3.125

[9] Darmstadta GL, Leea ACC, Cousensc S, Sibleyd L, Bhuttae ZA, Donnayb F, et al. 60 million non-facility births: Who can deliver in community settings to reduce intrapartum-related deaths? International Journal of Gynecology & Obstetrics. 2009;**107**:S89-S112. DOI: 10.1016/j.ijgo.2009.07.010

[10] Valentin D. Reducing maternal and child morbidity and mortality through project recommendations. [Doctoral study]. Walden University; 2016

[11] UNICEF. State of the World's Children 2009. New York: UNICEF; 2009

[12] Global Health Workforce Alliance. The 3rd Global Forum on Human Resources for Health. The Recife Political Declaration on Human Resources for Health: renewed commitments towards universal health coverage. Recife; 2013. Available from: http://www.who.int/workforcealliance/forum/2013/recife_declaration_17nov.pdf [Accessed: 23 August 2019]

[13] Taylor AL, Dhillon IS. The WHO global code of practice on the international recruitment of health personnel: The evolution of global health diplomacy. Global

Health Governance. 2011;**5**(1):1-24. Available from: https://scholarship.law.georgetown.edu/facpub/733 [Accessed: 23 August 2019]

[14] Brick A, Layte R, Nolan A, Turner MJ. Differences in nulliparous caesarean section rates across models of care: A decomposition analysis. BMC Health Services Research. 2016;**16**:239. DOI: 10.1186/s12913-016-1494-3

[15] Prah J, Kudom A, Afrifa A, Abdulai M, Sirikyi I, Abu E. Caesarean section in a primary health facility in Ghana: Clinical indications and feto-maternal outcomes. Journal of Public Health in Africa. 2017;**8**(704):155-159

[16] Higginbottom GMA, Safipour J, Mumtaz Z, Chiu Y, Paton P, Pillay J. "I have to do what I believe": Sudanese women's beliefs and resistance to hegemonic practices at home and during experiences of maternity care in Canada. BMC Pregnancy and Childbirth. 2013;**13**:51. DOI: 10.1186/1471-2393-13-51

[17] Leitch CR, Walker JJ. The rise in caesarean section rate: The same indications but a lower threshold. British Journal of Obstetrics and Gynaecology. 1998;**105**(6):621-626

[18] Surapanthapisit P, Thitadilok W. Risk factors of caesarean section due to cephalopelvic disproportion. Journal of the Medical Association of Thailand. 2006;**89**(Suppl 4):S105-S111. Available from: http://www.medassocthai.org/journal [Accessed: 25 August 2019]

[19] Mujugira A, Osoti A, Deya R, Hawes SE, Phipps AI. Fetal head circumference, operative delivery, and fetal outcomes: A multi-ethnic population-based cohort study. BMC Pregnancy and Childbirth. 2013;**13**:106. Available from: http://www.biomedcentral.com/1471-2393/13/106 [Accessed: 25 August 2019]

[20] Moni M, Thanganadar AT, Yesubaktan SJ. A study on obstetric profile of mothers undergoing primary caesarean section and their neonatal outcome in a tertiary care centre, South Kerala. International Journal of Biomedical and Advance Research. 2015;**6**(12):835-838. DOI: 10.7439/ijbar

[21] Blackard CS, Viera AJA. Retrospective review of performance and utility of routine clinical pelvimetry. Family Medicine. 2004;**36**(7):505-507

[22] Hofmeyr G. Obstructed labor : Using better technologies to reduce mortality. International Journal of Gynecology & Obstetrics. 2004;**85**:S62-S72

[23] Balleyguier C, Jouanic JM, Corréas JM, Benachi A, Dumez Y, Menu Y. CT pelvimetry: A new approach using multi detector CT and volume rendering. Journal de Radiologie. 2003 Apr;**84**(4 Pt 1):425-427

[24] Huerta-Enochian GS, Katz VL, Fox LK, Hamlin JA, Kollath JP. Magnetic resonance-based serial pelvimetry: Do maternal pelvic dimensions change during pregnancy? American Journal of Obstetrics and Gynecology. 2006 Jun;**194**(6):1689-1694; discussion 1694-5

[25] Liselele HB, Boulvain M, Tshibangu KC, Meuris S. Maternal height and external pelvimetry to predict cephalopelvic disproportion in nulliparous African women : A cohort study. BJOG: An International Journal of Obstetrics and Gynecology. 2000 Aug;**107**(8):947-952

[26] Rozenholc AT, Ako SN, Leke RJ, Boulvain M. The diagnostic accuracy of external pelvimetry and maternal height to predict dystocia in nulliparous women: A study in Cameroon. BJOG: An International Journal of

Obstetrics and Gynecology. 2007 May;**114**(5):630-635

[27] Kordi M, Alijahan R. The diagnostic accuracy of external pelvimetry to predict dystocia in nulliparous women. The Zahedan Journal of Research in Medical Sciences. 2012;**14**(6):36-38

[28] Alijahan R, Kordi M, Pourjavad P, Ebrahimzadeh S. Diagnostic accuracy of maternal anthropometric measurements as predictors for dystocia in nulliparous women. Iranian Journal of Nursing and Midwifery Research [Serial Online]. 2014;**19**:11-18. Available from: http://www.ijnmrjournal.net/text.asp?2014/19/1/11/124538 [cited 19 July 2019]

[29] Government of Rwanda. Health system. 14 Mar 2013. Available from: http://www.gov.rw/Health-System

[30] World Bank. Rwanda overview. 14 Mar 2013. Available from: http://www.worldbank.org/en/country/rwanda/overview

[31] Kakoma JB. Postgraduate and research programmes in medicine and public health in Rwanda: An exciting experience about training of human resources for health in a limited resources country. Pan African Medical Journal. 2016;**23**:171. DOI: 10.11604/pamj.2016.23.171.8788

[32] Coe NM, Kelly PF, Yeung HWC. Economic Geography : A contemporary Introduction. 2nd ed. Oxford: Blackwell; 2007

[33] Majoko F, Nyström L, Munjanja SP, Mason E, Lindmark G. Relation of parity to pregnancy outcome in a rural Community in Zimbabwe. African Journal of Reproductive Health. 2004;**8**(3):198-206

[34] Bai J, Wong FWS, Bauman A, Mohsin M. Parity and pregnancy outcomes. American Journal of Obstetrics and Gynecology. Feb 2002;**186**(2):274-278

[35] Kyembwa Mulyumba M, Juakali Sihalikyo KV, Katenga Bosunga G, Manga Okenge P, Kakoma Sakatolo JB. Risk Factors of Pre-eclampsia in Goma (Democratic Republic of the Congo). African Journal of Health Issues. 21 Aug 2018;**3**:12. DOI: 10.26875/ajhi232018xii

[36] Ashfaq M, Jabeen S, Hanif A. Frequency of Iron deficiency Anemia in nulliparous pregnant females during last trimester. Pakistan Journal of Medical and Health Sciences. Jan–Mar 2018;**12**(1):379-381

[37] Duckitt K, Harrington D. Risk factors for pre-eclampsia at antenatal booking: Systematic review of controlled studies. British Medical Journal. 2005;**330**:565. DOI: 10.1136/bmj.38380.674340.E0

[38] Christianson LM, Bovbjerg E, McDavitt EC, Hullfish L. Risk factors for perineal injury during delivery. American Journal of Obstetrics and Gynecology. July 2003;**189**(1):255-260

[39] Son Tran T, Silom Jamulitrat S, Chongsuvivatwong V, Geater A. Risk factors for postcesarean surgical site infection. Obstetrics & Gynecology. Mar 2000;**95**(3):367-371. DOI: 10.1016/S0029-7844(99)00540-2

[40] Shields SG, Ratcliffe SD, Fontaine P, Leeman L. Dystocia in nulliparous women. American Family Physician. 2007;**75**:1671-1678

[41] Mbukani R, JBSZ Kakoma. Is nulliparity a risk factor for poor obstetrical and neonatal outcomes in Rwandan district hospitals ? A prospective observational study at Muhima District Hospital. Rwanda Medical Journal. Mar 2012;**69**(1):50-53

[42] Bais JMJ, Eskes M, Pel M, Bonsel GJ, Bleker O. Postpartum haemorrhage in nulliparous women: Incidence and risk factors in low and high risk women. A Dutch population-based cohort study on standard (> or = 500 mL) and severe (> or = 1000 mL) postpartum haemorrhage. European Journal of Obstetrics & Gynecology and Reproductive Biology. Sep 2004;**115**(2):166-172

[43] Phupong V, Suebnukarn K. Obstetric outcomes in nulliparous young adolescent. The Southeast Asian Journal of Tropical Medicine and Public Health. Jan 2007;**38**(1):141-145

[44] Nyandekwe M, Nzayirambaho M, Kakoma JB. Universal health coverage in Rwanda: Dream or reality. The Pan African Medical Journal. 2014;**17**:232. DOI: 10.11604/pamj.2014.17.232.3471

[45] Nyandekwe M, Kakoma JB, Nzayirambaho M. The health-related millennium development goals (MDGs) 2015: Rwanda performance and contributing factors. The Pan African Medical Journal. 2018;**31**(56). DOI: 10.11604/pamj.2018.31.56.11018

[46] Semasaka Sengoma JP, Krantz G, Nzayirambaho M, Munyanshongore C, Edvardsson K, Mogren I. Prevalence of pregnancy-related complications and course of labour of surviving women who gave birth in selected health facilities in Rwanda: A health facility-based, cross-sectional study. BMJ Open. 2017;7:e015015. DOI: 10.1136/bmjopen-2016-01501

[47] Munan R, Yves Kakudji Y, Nsambi J, Mukuku O, Maleya A, Kinenkinda X, et al. Accouchement chez la primipare à Lubumbashi: pronostic maternel et périnatal. Pan African Medical Journal. 2017;**28**(77). DOI: 10.11604/pamj.2017.28.77.1371

[48] Villar J, Valladares E, Wojdyla D, Zavaleta N, Carroli G, et al. Caesarean delivery rates and pregnancy outcomes: The 2005 WHO global survey on maternal and perinatal health in Latin America. Lancet. 2006;**367**(9525):1819-1829

[49] Althabe F, Sosa C, Belizán JM, Gibbons L, Jacquerioz F, et al. Cesarean section rates and maternal and neonatal mortality in low-, medium-, and high-income countries: An ecological study. Birth. 2006;**33**(4):270-277

[50] Human Reproduction Programme. WHO Statement on Caesarean Section Rates. Geneva: World Health Organization; 2015

[51] Soto-Vega E, Casco S, Chamizo K, Flores-Hernández D, Landini V, Guillén-Florez A. Rising trends of cesarean section worldwide: A systematic review. Obstetrics and Gynecology International Journal. 2015;**3**(2):00073. DOI: 10.15406/ogij.2015.03.00073

[52] Soumya RP, Madhu J, Shuchi J. Rising trend in Caesarean section rate: A community health hazard. Biomedical Journal of Scientific & Technical Research. 2017;**1**(5):1476-1479. DOI: 10.26717/BJSTR.2017.01.000464

[53] Kagaba A. Incidence, indications, and outcome of cesarean section at King Faisal Hospital, Kigali (2005-2006). [MD dissertation]. National University of Rwanda; 2006

[54] Mugarura JC. Aspects épidémiologiques et cliniques des césariennes pratiquées en 2006 à la Maternité de l'Hôpital de Byumba. [MD dissertation]. National University of Rwanda; 2007

[55] Kakoma JB. Cesarean section indications and anthropometric parameters in Rwandan nulliparae: Preliminary results from a longitudinal survey. Pan African Medical Journal.

2016;**24**:310. DOI: 10.11604/pamj.2016.24.310.9603

[56] Kinenkinda X, Mukuku O, Chenge F, Kakudji P, Banzulu P, Kakoma JB, et al. Césarienne à Lubumbashi, République Démocratique du Congo I: fréquence, indications et mortalité maternelle et périnatale. Pan African Medical Journal. 2017;**27**(72). DOI: 10.11604/pamj.2017.27.72.1214

[57] Kakoma SZJB. Histoire de la Gynécologie-Obstétrique. Presses Universitaires de Lubumbashi. Lubumbashi; 1998

[58] Kakoma SZJB. Pelvis and anthropometric study in Rwandan women at prenatal care in the Southern Province of Rwanda (Huye District). Rwanda Medical Journal. Mar 2010;**69**:13-25

[59] Kalibushi JB. Pelvis study in Rwandan women at prenatal care clinics or delivery room and its obstetrical implications in urban area (Kigali city). [MMed/OG dissertation]. National University of Rwanda; 2010

[60] Malonga FK. Anthropométrie et pelvimétrie clinique externe des gestantes de Lubumbashi: Déterminants de Prédiction de la voie d'accouchement. [Thèse d'Agrégation de l'enseignement supérieur en médecine]. Université de Lubumbashi; 2018

[61] Kakoma JBSZ, Kalibushi J, Ramazani KR. Height, weight, external pelvic diameters and cesarean section: A cohort study in Southern Province of Rwanda (Huye District). Rwanda Medical Journal. Sep 2010;**68**(3):21-24

[62] Ngoy JK. Mesures de la base du triangle de Trillat et du diamètre bi-ischiatique : Relations entre les paramètres mesurés et l'issue obstétricale chez la nullipare à Lubumbashi. [Mémoire de spécialisation en gynécologie—obstétrique]. Université de Lubumbashi; 2018

[63] Ngalula MT. Le dépistage de la disproportion céphalo-pelvienne chez la nullipare à Lubumbashi (RD Congo): Apport de la pelvimétrie externe et des mensurations de la hauteur utérine et de la taille maternelle. [Mémoire de spécialisation en gynécologie—obstétrique]. Université de Lubumbashi; 2018

[64] Malonga FK, Mukuku O, Ngalula MT, Kakudji PL, Kakoma JB. Étude anthropométrique et pelvimétrique externe chez les nullipares de Lubumbashi: facteurs de risque et score prédictif de la dystocie mécanique. Pan African Medical Journal. 2018;**31**:69. DOI: 10.11604/pamj.2018.31.69.16014

[65] Kumar S, Vatsa R, Bharti J, Roy KK, Sharma JB, Singh N, et al. Urinary fistula—A continuing problem with changing trends. Journal of the Turkish-German Gynecological Association. 2017 Mar;**18**(1):15-19. DOI: 10.4274/jtgga.2016.0211

[66] Eilber KS, Kavaler E, Rodriguiz LV, Rosenblum N, Raz S. Ten-year experience with transvaginal vesicovaginal fistula repair using tissue interposition. The Journal of Urology. 2003;**169**:1033-1036

[67] Cowgill KD, Bishop J, Norgaard AK. Obstetric fistula in low-resource countries: An under-valued and under-studied problem—Systematic review of its incidence, prevalence, and association with stillbirth. BMC Pregnancy and Childbirth. 2015;**15**:193

[68] Nsambi JB, Mukuku O, Foma JDY, Kinenkinda X, Kakudji P, Kizonde J, et al. Fistules obstétricales dans la province du Haut-Katanga, République Démocratique du Congo: à propos de 242 cas. Pan African Medical Journal. 2018;**29**:34. DOI: 10.11604/pamj.2018.29.34.14576

Chapter 6

# Quality Care for Mothers and Newborns at Birth in Mexico

*Bonifacio Caballero Noguéz, Roberto Aguli Ruíz Rosas and Ernesto Calderon Cisneros*

## Abstract

Estimates of the United Nations (UN) consider that in the world 2.5 million neonates died in the last year from preventable causes such as prematurity, complications during childbirth, and infections. Some died because the care they received was of poor quality. The most striking is that 1.7 million newborns could be saved by improving access to quality care for all pregnant women in humanitarian settings, especially those considered as low- and middle-income countries by the World Bank. Neonatal mortality can be considered as a sensitive indicator of the well-being of a population, the degree of development of a country, as well as health conditions in the mother's environment and the good quality of prenatal and intrapartum care. This will seek the achievement of the Sustainable Development Goals (SDGs) of the United Nations, through universal health coverage (UHC), by 2030. The medical advances that obstetrics has had around history show the interest and importance for the health sector of all countries in the world, the attention of women, especially during the reproductive stage in which it is located at stake the life and health of the human capital of the future. Today, obstetrics is the health science recognized worldwide because it addresses the health of women during the preconception, conception, prenatal, childbirth, postnatal, and postconception stages, as well as the newborn. Every day more progress is made, not only in the increasingly early diagnosis, but also in the care, attention during the months of gestation, and studies and tests to be carried out to have a greater certainty of what happens inside the uterus-definitely, we are going forward. But the latter is not available to all pregnant women, or in all regions of Mexico, because of the asymmetry in the structure, with imbalance in qualified human resources and technology that detract from this quality of care that is intended. Therefore, we are still reporting preventable maternal deaths and preterm infants, and the interest of this chapter is to show the need, as referred by the World Health Organization (WHO), to improve the quality of care with qualified personnel: obstetricians for women and neonatologists or pediatricians for newborn care.

**Keywords:** childbirth, birth care, newborn, prematurity, sustainable development goals, Mexico

## 1. Introduction

"There is no concept of normalcy during labour and childbirth." Because complications that increase morbidity and mortality of the mother-child binomial may occur during the process.

In 2015, the United Nations Organization (UN) established Agenda 2030 for Sustainable Development Goals (SDGs) as an action plan for people, where it highlights the importance of measures to ensure maternal and child health.

Under the SDGs, specifically, SDG 3 sets targets for 2030 to reduce maternal mortality rates below 70 per 100,000 live births and neonatal mortality for all countries to no more than 12 per 1000 live births [1].

Achieving this will require effective strategies and targeted actions, as well as monitoring progress against basic indicators of maternal and child health (MCH). In this regard, one of the key indicators, which is explicitly adopted in the SDGs and the Global Strategy for Women's, Children's and Adolescents' Health 2016–2030, is the proportion of births attended by skilled health personnel [2].

This approach is aimed at preventing the highest number of preventable deaths, including mothers, fetuses, and newborns.

## 2. Preterm birth is a syndrome

Premature childbirth should be considered a syndrome by the multiple processes that trigger it, some pathological and others still unknown [3].

In essence, both the beginning of term labor and premature delivery share a similar clinical process: increased uterine contractility, cervical dilation, and rupture of the chorioamniotic membranes [3].

However, despite efforts to reduce these risk factors, the rate of preterm births continues to rise.

Intra-amniotic infection has been causally associated with premature delivery [4].

One third of newborns have the history that their mother has, which is an intra-amniotic infection from the association of isolated germs in the amniotic fluid and the similarity of those found in the genital tract. Similarly, bacteria have been found involved in periodontal pathology, suggesting the possibility of hematogenous dissemination and transplacental passage, although the ascending pathway is considered the most frequent route of infection. Since bacteria have been found in the circulation of premature patients, it suggests that there is a systemic inflammatory response (infection/inflammation) [5, 6].

The microbiological diagnosis of an intra-amniotic infection has been based on the use of culture techniques (adequate nutritional and environmental conditions) with the growth of bacteria obtained from the amniotic fluid.

The theory that describes the biofilm process described in 1978 states that bacteria grow in communities called "biofilms," which generally adhere to surfaces, and that most bacteria grow in biofilms enclosed within a matrix, so they differ from their isolated forms observed in Gram staining tests of biological fluids or pure cultures (planktonics, so named for their similar shape to marine plankton) [7].

Biofilms are now recognized as playing an important role in human diseases.

Infections outside the genitourinary area such as periodontitis, otitis media, endocarditis, and many others where there is a device (prosthetic valves or catheters) involve bacterial biofilms [8].

In view of this possibility, molecular microbiological techniques have recently been used to detect microorganisms in the amniotic cavity [9].

On the other hand, about 25% of premature newborns are born as a result of a medical intervention to interrupt pregnancy when complications such as preeclampsia or maternal comorbidity occurs (heart disease and systemic lupus erythematosus, among others) [10].

Approximately 50% of all premature births are due to unknown causes or multifactorial processes that cause the uterus to move from a state of inactivity to one of active contractions. In other words spontaneous premature delivery of unknown etiology can be initiated in up to half of the cases by multiple causes (gene-gene and gene-environmental interactions, such as smoking cigarettes, short cervix, young maternal age, assisted reproduction technology (overdistension of the uterus caused by multiple pregnancy), socioeconomic and cultural aspects that condition late or nonprenatal care, and previous premature delivery) [11–15].

## 3. World situation

It is estimated that approximately 140 million births occur annually in the world, in women without risk factors or comorbidity to present complications for both them and their babies, at the beginning and during labor [16].

However, in addition to the possible complications that can occur during labor, there is the problem related to premature delivery that occurs between 5 and 18% of pregnancies and is one of the main causes of morbidity and mortality in the neonatal stage.

Premature newborns are at increased risk of short-term complications attributed to organic immaturity, especially at the central nervous system level with neurodevelopmental disorders such as cerebral palsy and intellectual, visual, and auditory disabilities [17].

Therein lies the importance for the prevention and treatment of premature labor and thus to remain under the goals of the SDGs [18].

It is estimated that approximately 15 million births will be premature (11%), half of which will be due to unknown or unclear causes [19–21].

In recent decades, advances in neonatal care have been significant and there are reports of survival of newborns with gestational age from 22 weeks (22–26 weeks, a period commonly considered "periviable").

In particular, pregnant women considered to be at high risk of periviable childbirth have been treated in tertiary care hospitals with neonatal intensive care units (NICUs) level 3 [22].

For this reason, reducing the rate of premature births requires a better understanding of the mechanisms responsible.

The mechanism that determines the beginning of the term or preterm birth is not known, although it is considered multifactorial.

In recent years, premature childbirth has increased globally, becoming a problem in obstetric care and one of the main causes of infant death worldwide, a serious problem for health systems. Premature birth accounts for more than 85% of all complications and perinatal deaths during the infant stage [23].

Morbidity, early mortality, and the presence of lifelong sequelae of a premature newborn will depend to a large extent on the country where he or she is born. In countries considered low income, disability problems are rare, particularly in newborns under 28 weeks of pregnancy or those with some pathology [24].

They die because of lack of adequate prenatal care or medical care with infrastructure and qualified personnel. In middle-income countries, newborns born between 28 and 33 weeks of gestation have improved the prognosis of survival but will have almost twice as many disability problems as those from high-income countries. In high-income countries, more than 95% survive with lower morbidity and sequelae [25].

Alternatives that can be applied, safe and available in all countries to prevent premature delivery, mainly before 34 weeks of gestation, should therefore be investigated [26].

Improvement in health care for women, children, and adolescents is included in the SDGs, which aim to ensure that the mother-children not only survive the complications that may occur during childbirth but also achieve the maximum potential in health [27, 28].

It is important to emphasize that public health policies implemented to protect the binomial do not have to be specific; they must guarantee the quality of care, because there are differences in the world related to the infrastructure and quantity of human resources in the care services that are available for each country or region. And, they include the care of labor, labor, expulsion period, delivery, and resuscitation of the newborn and the mother after delivery [29].

## 4. Friendly obstetric care

Historically, birth was considered a natural process imbued with a strong cultural and social context, before its care and care by medical personnel was initiated, with what was modified the roles where the mother and the newborn had the leading role, becoming an "impersonal" process and often alien to their sociocultural condition, pathologizing pregnancy and especially labor, with abuse at times of medicalization [30, 31].

It is also important not only to identify but also to eradicate cultural barriers that hinder access to health services, because of the cultural and economic diversity that can exist among the population. In many countries, traditional and professional midwifery has emerged as an alternative to unconventional therapeutic models [32, 33].

In recent decades, a number of practices relating to labor have been increasingly developed with the aim of initiating to accelerate, finish, regulate, or monitor what should be considered a physiological process in order to achieve better results for the binomial [34–40].

While these have contributed to decreasing maternal and perinatal morbi-mortality, in countries with low and medium incomes, they promote the use of unnecessary interventions and neglect the emotional needs of pregnant women, leaving the mother to play a secondary role and contributing to the increase in the overall cost of medical services [41].

The gap in maternal and perinatal deaths is disproportionate between low- and middle-income countries compared to high-income countries [42].

It can also generate a perception, in women, of being excluded during their care by not having a participation in decision-making in the performance of some procedures.

Therefore, improving the quality of care around the time of birth, especially in low- and medium-income countries, has been identified as the most striking strategy for reducing fetal deaths and maternal and neonatal deaths, compared to prenatal or postpartum care strategies [26].

Mexico ranks fourth in the world (after China, Brazil, and the United States) in the use of cesarean sections without medical indication (38.5% of births); this percentage is above the World Health Organization (WHO) recommendation that the percentage of births per cesarean section should not exceed 15% [43].

WHO has proposed the model of friendly obstetric care. The pleasant and human experience of childbirth must nowadays be the desire of all women and also the goal of all doctors, especially obstetricians [44].

This is used as a strategy to reduce maternal morbidity by explicitly and directly taking back the emotional needs and values of women and their families in the care of pregnancy and birth and during puerperium, emphasizing the intercultural aspects that recognize the diversity that exists among women, and in order to eradicate cultural barriers by promoting the right to scientific health care by health professionals who have the best obstetric skills, focusing on pregnant women empowering them to make decisions and returning them to their leading role [45].

## 5. "Support" for women during childbirth

### 5.1 Description of the condition

From the dawn of history and between different cultures, women were cared for and supported by other women during labor and childbirth, which has been called "continuous support," excluding the "man" during practically the labor, delivery, and birth of the baby.

However, since the middle of the nineteenth century, in many countries, especially in Europe, a large percentage of pregnant women had their births in hospital rather than at home.

Until Ignaz Philipp Semmelweis (Allgemeines Krankenhaus der Stadt Wien) in 1847 proposed to wash his hands, as the puerperal fever caused the death of 10–35%, which was three to five times higher than those attended by "midwives" is the word. Consequently, continued support during childbirth became the exception rather than the norm.

At the beginning of this century, the experiences of childbirth in women (especially in high-, middle-, and low-income countries) have led to the resumption of individual support for women during childbirth [46].

Recent publications show that many women benefit from and value the presence of a support person during childbirth, which provides them with psychological, physical, emotional, informative, and practical support, respecting their interculturality and privacy [47].

WHO recommends the presence of a companion of choice of woman during childbirth [48, 49].

In this same perspective, the aim is to "oversell" the care of low-risk childbirth. It is described in the literature as a highly medicalized care model that promotes the use of unnecessary interventions, neglects the emotional needs of pregnant women, promotes cesarean section intervention, and contributes to the increase in the overall cost of medical services [41].

In hospitals in middle-income countries, especially in Latin America, women in labor are without support and under a model of medicalized care [50].

This model of care is carried out mainly in urban areas, where more than 70% of the population currently resides.

## 6. Obstetric care in Mexico

In Mexico, more than 90% of women living in large cities have their births in hospitals, with a high number of unnecessary practices of little scientific value, such as trichotomy, amnesty, indiscriminate use of ocytocytics, episiotomies, and cesarean sections, indicators of a high level of medicalization [34, 38, 39, 41, 51].

The ratios of maternal mortality in countries such as Mexico in 2018 were 34 cases per 100,000 live births, with variations among the different federal entities, suggesting that many of the causes of maternal mortality are preventable [52].

In teenage girls, the risk of complications during pregnancy, childbirth, or puerperium has a greater impact.

In the period from 2004 to 2009, 8.6% of pregnancies ended in abortion, making it the 5th leading cause of maternal deaths.

In the last 12 years, the medicalized model has become a public health problem since approximately 50.3% of the births by women aged 20–49 years were obtained by cesarean section. Only 25.7% had emergency medical indication. The highest number is in private care institutions with 60.4% of the total [53–56].

Although efforts are being made to overemphasize the care of labor in childbirth and to reduce the percentage of cesarean sections to the figures recommended by WHO (15%), progress in this regard is slow [57, 58].

If prenatal care does not meet quality standards, the chances of a large number of pregnant women ending up with premature delivery are high. It is where cultural factors and social and economic conditions will influence its presence.

The institution where the authors work Mexican Social Security Institute (Instituto Mexicano del Seguro Social, IMSS) provides social security to more than 50% of the Mexican population.

**Figure 1** shows the trend of the maternal mortality ratio recorded in the last 17 years in Mexico (upper line). In the lower line of the graph is the reason that corresponds to the IMSS during the same period.

The safety approach includes the obstetric skills that the first contact staff must have for identifying obstetric risks during pregnancy, as well as for delivery care in accordance with the recommendations of WHO and for the management and referral of complications of WHO. With regard to the level of the hospital, it should have all the competences, conditions, and interinstitutional agreements, in order to be able to identify, attend to, and resolve obstetric complications and emergencies in a timely manner, within a strategy of real functional flow networks in health services, to ensure timely care for women in labor, with or without complications, under the "zero rejection" initiative [59].

Each country should develop strategies to improve access to care, in line with different health care systems. In Mexico, there are several social security systems (public) to try to guarantee the health of its population, leaving a very low percentage of the population without social security coverage and those who have the possibility of being cared for in private institutions [60].

In Mexico, the "Comprehensive Interinstitutional Partnership Agreement for Obstetric Emergencies" was developed to provide immediate medical care to women in the severe puerperal period, with an emergency that endangers their lives, where care for newborns is also included.

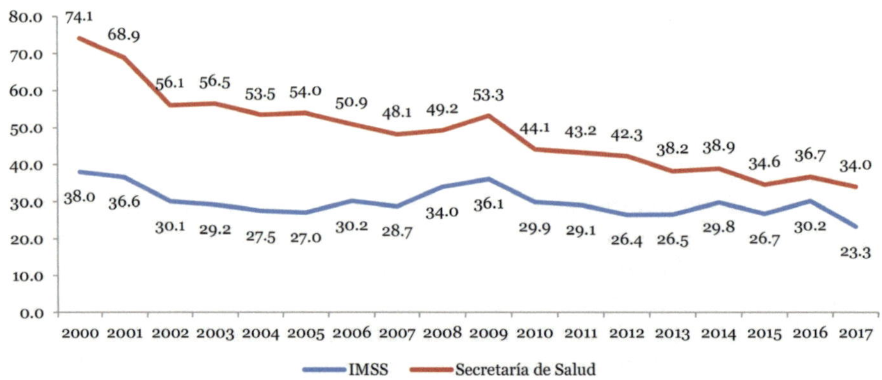


**Figure 1.**
*Maternal mortality ratio in Mexico (2000–2017). *Source: Secretaria de Salud and Instituto Mexicano del Seguro Social.*

This agreement is a written agreement between the health institutions that set out the general guidelines for the medical units of the SS of the Institute for Social Security and Services of State Workers (ISSSTE) and the Mexican Social Security Institute (IMSS), with capacity for complex obstetric care by providing these services through immediate response teams, to women with an obstetric emergency.

**Table 1** shows the top 10 causes of hospital discharge in IMSS. It is noted that obstetric care (pregnancy, childbirth, and puerperium), while not being an illness, was the first reason for hospital discharge, representing 25% (517,800) of total discharges, in the period from July 2018 to June 2019.

| **Causes** | | **Discharges** | |
|---|---|---|---|
| | | **Thousands** | **%** |
| 1 | Pregnancy, childbirth, and the puerperium | 517.8 | 25 |
| 2 | Injuries and poisonings | 164.8 | 8 |
| 3 | Heart diseases | 97.4 | 5 |
| 4 | Malignant tumors | 91.4 | 4 |
| 5 | Cholelithiasis and cholecystitis | 85.6 | 4 |
| 6 | Renal insufficiency | 85.0 | 4 |
| 7 | Conditions originating in the perinatal period | 72.3 | 3 |
| 8 | Diabetes mellitus | 55.5 | 3 |
| 9 | Hernias | 41.2 | 2 |
| 10 | Pneumonia and influenza | 40.7 | 2 |
| **Sum of the 10 main causes** | | **1251.0** | **59** |
| **Total** | | **2112.3** | **100** |

*The numbers from March to June 2019 were calculated. Source: IMSS.*

**Table 1.**
*The 10 main hospital discharge in the Mexican Social Security Institute (July 2018 to June 2019).*

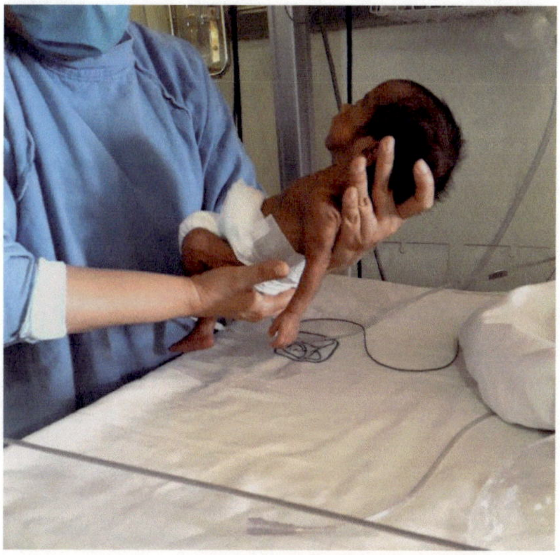

**Figure 2.**
*A premature newborn treated at IMSS, from the "early intervention" program.*

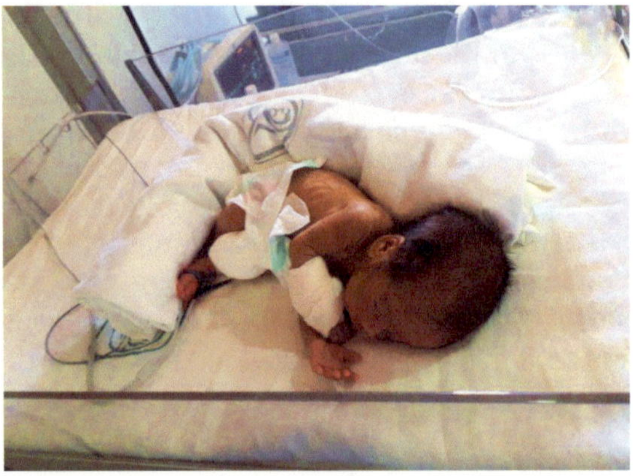

**Figure 3.**
*A premature newborn treated in IMSS close to his hospital discharge.*

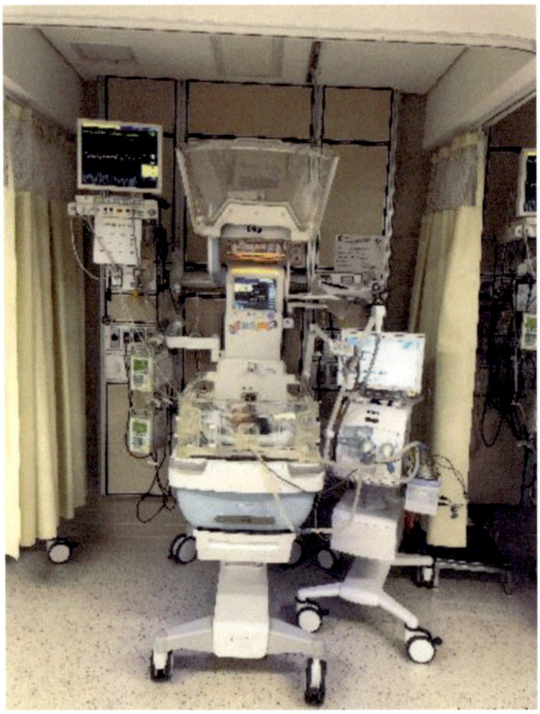

**Figure 4.**
*The economic cost and technological equipment required in the care of the premature newborn.*

The IMSS serves almost 50% of all public sector births in the country. In 2017, 425,516 births were registered; of these, 9.8% (41,664) were premature under 37 weeks of gestational age and 7320 (1.7%) weighed less than 1500 g.

In **Figures 2–4**, we show preterm newborns treated in IMSS.

## 7. Conclusions

Measures to contain prematurity should essentially aim at improving the quality of pregnancy care. In countries such as Mexico, it is necessary to define, in addition to what we described, the measures that impact to reduce premature delivery due to avoidable conditions.

Despite all measures for monitoring and care, the rate of premature births in the world has risen steadily. Medical efforts should be directed at improving results in the care of premature newborns and diminishing the impact on the neurodevelopment of infant and their families, as they would represent a high social impact and economic cost.

It would be advisable to prolong premature births to 34–36 weeks of gestation in order to reduce infant mortality, especially in medium- and low-income countries. This measure would significantly benefit from and would make reasonable use of the highly specialized technological and human resources that are usually limited.

What are needed are prevention, prenatal surveillance with a risk approach, and care during childbirth and of the newborn with qualified personnel, and current research is directed toward achieving this goal.

## Author details

Bonifacio Caballero Noguéz, Roberto Aguli Ruíz Rosas*
and Ernesto Calderon Cisneros
Social Security Mexican Institute (IMSS), Mexico City, Mexico

*Address all correspondence to: rruizrosas@gmail.com

## References


[1] Sustainable Development Goals. Available from: https://sustainabledevelopment.un.org/?menu=1300

[2] The Global Strategy for Women's, Children's and Adolescents' Health, 2016-2030. Available from: http://www.who.int/life-course/partners/global-strategy/global-strategy-2016-2030/en/

[3] Romero R, Espinoza J, Kusanovic JP, Gotsch F, et al. The preterm parturition syndrome. BJOG. 2006;**113**(Suppl 3):17-42

[4] Romero R, Gómez R, Chaiworapongsa T, Conoscenti G, et al. The role of infection in preterm labour and delivery. Paediatric and Perinatal Epidemiology. 2001;**15**(Suppl 2):41-56

[5] Carroll SG, Ville Y, Greenough A, Gamsu H, et al. Preterm prelabour amniorrhexis: Intrauterine infection and interval between membrane rupture and delivery. Archives of Disease in Childhood. Fetal and Neonatal Edition. 1995;**72**(1):F43-F46

[6] Gómez R, Romero R, Ghezzi F, Yoon BH, et al. The fetal inflammatory response syndrome. American Journal of Obstetrics and Gynecology. 1998;**179**(1):194-202

[7] Costerton JW, Geesey GG, Cheng KJ. How bacteria stick. Scientific American. 1978;**238**(1):86-95

[8] Costerton JW, Stewart PS, Greenberg EP. Bacterial biofilms: A common cause of persistent infections. Science. 1999;**284**(5418):1318-1322

[9] Gardella C, Riley DE, Hitti JK, Agnew JN, Krieger D. Eschenbach identification and sequencing of bacterial rDNAs in culture-negative amniotic fluid from women in premature labor. American Journal of Perinatology. 2004;**21**:319-323

[10] Bennett P, Thornton S. Preterm birth. Best Practice & Research. Clinical Obstetrics & Gynaecology. 2007;**21**:727-728

[11] March of Dimes, PMNCH, Save the Children, WHO. In: Howson CP, Kinney MV, Lawn JE, editors. Born Too Soon: The Global Action Report on Preterm Birth. Geneva, Switzerland: World Health Organization; 2012

[12] Rubens C, Sadovsky Y, Muglia L, Gravett M, Lackritz E, Gravett C. Prevention of preterm birth: Harnessing science to address the global epidemic. Science Translational Medicine. 2015;**6**:262sr5

[13] Romero R, Dey SK, Fisher S. Preterm labor: One syndrome, many causes. Science. 2014;**345**:760-765

[14] Behrman RE, Butler AS, editors. Preterm Birth: Causes, Consequences, and Prevention. Institute of Medicine (US) Committee on Understanding Premature Birth and Assuring Healthy Outcomes. Washington, DC: National Academies Press (US); 2007

[15] Menon R, Bonney E. Oxidative stress and premature delivery. In: Dennery PA, Buonocore G, Saugstad OD, editors. Perinatal and Prenatal. New York: Springer; 2014. pp. 95-115

[16] Hamilton JG, Lobel M. Psychosocial factors associated with risk perceptions for chronic diseases in younger and middle-aged women. Women & Health. 2015;**55**(8):921-942. DOI: 10.1080/03630242.2015.1061094

[17] Mwaniki MK, Atieno M, Lawn JE, Newton CR. Long-term neurodevelopmental outcomes after

intrauterine and neonatal insults: A systematic review. Lancet. 2012;**379**:445

[18] Liu L, Oza S, Hogan D, Chu Y, Perin J, Zhu J, et al. Global, regional, and national causes of under-5 mortality in 2000-15: An updated systematic analysis with implications for the sustainable development goals. Lancet. 2016;**388**(10063):3027-3035

[19] Schober L, Radnai D, Schmitt E, Mahnke K, Sohn C, Steinborn A. Term and preterm labor: Decreased suppressive activity and changes in composition of the regulatory T-cell pool. Immunology and Cell Biology. 2012;**90**:935-944

[20] Novak TE, Babcock TA, Jho DH, Helton WS, Espat NJ. NF-kappa B inhibition by omega −3 fatty acids modulates LPS-stimulated macrophage TNF-alpha transcription. American Journal of Physiology-Lung Cellular and Molecular Physiology. 2003;**284**:L84-L89

[21] Martínez FO, Helming L, Gordon S. Alternative activation of macrophages: An immunologic functional perspective. Annual Review of Immunology. 2009;**27**:451-483

[22] Tyson JE, Parikh NA, Langer J, Green C, Higgins RD. Intensive care for extreme prematurity—Moving beyond gestational age. The New England Journal of Medicine. 2008;**358**:1672-1681

[23] Vogel JP, Chawanpaiboon S, Watananirun K, Lumbiganon P, Petzold M. Cols. Global, regional and national levels and trends of preterm birth rates for 1990 to 2014: Protocol for development of World Health Organization estimates. Reproductive Health. 2016;**13**(1):76. DOI: 10.1186/s12978-016-0193-1.

[24] Chawanpaiboon S, Vogel JP, Moller AB, Lumbiganon P, Petzold M. Global, regional, and national estimates of levels of preterm birth in 2014: A systematic review and modelling analysis. The Lancet Global Health. 2019;**7**(1):e37-e46. DOI: 10.1016/S2214-109X(18)30451-0

[25] Saigal S, Doyle LW. An overview of mortality and sequelae of preterm birth from infancy to adulthood. Lancet. 2008;**371**:261-269

[26] Bhutta ZA, Das JK, Bahl R, Lawn JE, Salam RA, Paul VK, et al. Can available interventions end preventable deaths in mothers, newborn babies, and stillbirths, and at what cost? Lancet. 2014;**384**:347-370

[27] WHO et al. Averting maternal death and disability. In: Monitoring Emergency Obstetric Care. A Handbook. Geneva: World Health Organization; 2009. Available from: http://www.who.int/reproductivehealth/publications/monitoring/9789241547734/en/ [Accessed: 02 June 2019]

[28] Every Woman Every Child. UN Commission on Life-Saving Commodities for Women and Children [website]. United Nations Foundation; 2012. Available from: http://everywomaneverychild.org/resources/un-commission-on-life-saving-commodities [Accessed: 01 May 2019]

[29] World Health Organization. Standards for improving quality of maternal and newborn care in health facilities. Available from: www.who.int/maternalchildadolescent/documents/improving-maternal-newborn-care-quality/en/ [Accessed: 05 May 2019]

[30] Sen G, Reddy B, Iyer A. Beyond measurement. The drivers of disrespect and abuse in obstetric care. Reproductive Health Matters. 2018;**26**(53):6-18. DOI: 10.1080/09688080.2018.1508173

[31] Azhar Z, Oyebode O, Masud H. Disrespect and abuse during childbirth in district Gujrat, Pakistan: A quest for respectful maternity care. PLoS One. 2018;**13**(7):e0200318. DOI: 10.1371/journal.pone.0200318. eCollection 2018

[32] Keleher KC. Collaborative practice. Characteristics, barriers, benefits, and implications for midwifery. Journal of Nurse-Midwifery. 1998;**43**:8e11

[33] Wallace HJ, McDonald S, Belton S, Miranda AI, da Costa E, et al. The decision to seek care antenatally and during labour and birth—who and what influences this in Timor-Leste? A qualitative project exploring the perceptions of Timorese women and men. Midwifery. 2018;**65**:35-42. DOI: 10.1016/j.midw.2018.05.013

[34] Jiang H, Qian X, Carroli G, Garner P. Selective versus routine use of episiotomy for vaginal birth. Cochrane Database of Systematic Reviews. 2017;**2**:CD000081. DOI: 10.1002/14651858.CD000081.pub3.

[35] Lawrence A, Lewis L, Hofmeyr GJ, Dowswell T, Styles C. Maternal positions and mobility during first stage labour. Cochrane Database of Systematic Reviews. 2013;**8**:CD003934

[36] Smyth RM, Markham C, Dowswell T. Amniotomy for shortening spontaneous labour. Cochrane Database of Systematic Reviews. 2013;**6**:CD006167

[37] Cuervo LG, Rodriguez MN, Delgado MB. Enemas during labor. Cochrane Database of Systematic Reviews. 2000;**2**:CD000330

[38] Kovavisarach E, Jirasettasiri P. Randomised controlled trial of perineal shaving versus hair cutting in parturients on admission in labor. Journal of the Medical Association of Thailand. 2005;**88**:1167e71

[39] Basevi V, Lavender T. Routine perineal shaving on admission in labour. Cochrane Database of Systematic Reviews. 2001;**1**:CD001236

[40] Singata M, Tranmer J, Gyte GM. Restricting oral fluid and food intake during labour. Cochrane Database of Systematic Reviews. 2010;**1**:CD003930

[41] Tracy SK, Tracy MB. Costing the cascade: Estimating the cost of increased obstetric intervention in childbirth using population data. BJOG. 2003;**110**(8):717-724

[42] WHO et al. Trends in Maternal Mortality: 1990-2013. Geneva: World Health Organization; 2014. Available from: http://www.who.int/reproductivehealth/publications/monitoring/maternalmortality-2013/en/ [Accessed: 12 June 2019]

[43] González-Pérez GJ, Vega López MG, Cabrera Pivaral CE. Cesáreas en México: Aspectos sociales, económicos y epidemiológicos. Universidad de Guadalajara, Centro Universitario de Ciencias de la Salud. 2011. Available from: http://www.cucs.udg.mx/revistas/libros/CESAREAS_EN_MEXICO_ASPECTOS_SOCIALES_ECONOMICOS_Y_EPIDEMIOLOGICOS.pdf

[44] Li Y-P, Yeh C-H, Lin S-Y, Chen T-C, Yang Y-L, Lee C-N, et al. A proposed mother-friendly childbirth model for Taiwanese women, the implementation and satisfaction survey. Taiwanese Journal of Obstetrics & Gynecology. 2015;**54**:731-736

[45] WHO. WHO Recommendations: Intrapartum Care for a Positive Childbirth Experience. Geneva: World Health Organization; 2018

[46] Klaus MH, Kennell JH, Klaus PH. The Doula Book: How a

Trained Labor Companion Can Help you Have a Shorter, Easier and Healthier Birth. 2nd ed. Cambridge, MA: Perseus Books; 2002

[47] Kabakian-Khasholian T, El-Nemer A, Bashour H. Perceptions about labor companionship at public teaching hospitals in three Arab countries. International Journal of Gynaecology and Obstetrics. 2015 Jun;**129**(3):223-226

[48] World Health Organization. Standards for improving quality of maternal and newborn care in health facilities. Available from: www.who.int/maternalchildadolescent/documents/improving-maternal-newborn-care-quality/en/ [Accessed: 25 June 2019]

[49] WHO Reproductive Health Library. Labour companionship: Every woman's choice. Available from: extranet.who.int/rhl/resources/videos/labour-companionship-every-womanschoice [Accessed: 25 June 2019]

[50] Savage V, Castro A. Measuring mistreatment of women during childbirth: A review of terminology and methodological approaches. Reproductive Health. 2017;**14**(1):138. DOI: 10.1186/s12978-017-0403-5

[51] Consejo Nacional de Evaluación de la Política de Desarrollo Social. Informe de Evaluación de la Política de Desarrollo Social. 2018

[52] Morales-AndradeE,Ayala-HernádezMI, Morales-ValerdiHF,Astorga-CastañedaM, Castro-Herrera GA. Epidemiología de la muerte materna en México y el cumplimiento del Objetivo 5 del Desarrollo del Milenio, hacia los objetivos de desarrollo sostenible. Revista de especialidades médico-quirúrgicas. 2018;**23**:61-86

[53] Puentes-Rosas E, Gómez-Dantés O, Garrido-Latorre F. Las cesáreas en México: tendencias, niveles y factores asociados. Salud Pública de México, [S.l.], v. 46, n. 1, pp. 16-22, ene. 2004. Available from: http://saludpublica.mx/index.php/spm/article/view/6507/7968 [Accessed: 26 June 2019]

[54] Instituto Nacional de Estadistica y Geografía (México). Mujeres y hombres en México. 2018. Instituto Nacional de Estadistica y Geografía. México: INEGI. 2018

[55] Secretaria de salud. Lineamiento técnico para la Cesárea segura. México. Centro Nacional de Equidad de Género y Salud Reproductiva. SSa. 2013

[56] Fonseca-Pérez J. Cesárea por solicitud materna (CPSM). Revista Colombiana de Obstetricia y Ginecología. 2017;**68**(1):7

[57] Instituto Mexicano de Seguro social. Guía de Práctica Clínica para la Reducción de la Frecuencia de Operación Cesárea. Evidencias y recomendaciones. Rev. IMSS Mexico [Internet]. 2014. Available from: www.cenetec.salud.gob.mx/interior/g pc.html

[58] Instituto Nacional de Salud Pública. Elevada recurrencia a las cesáreas: revertir la tendencia y mejorar la calidad en el parto. ENSANUT [Internet]. 2012. Available from: http://ensanut.insp.mx

[59] World Health Organization. Care in normal birth: A practical guide. Technical working group, World Health Organization. Birth. 1997;**24**:121-123

[60] Gutierrez JP, García-Saisó S, Fajardo Dolci G, Hernández Avila M. Effective access to health care in Mexico. BMC Health Services Research. 2014;**14**(1):186. DOI: 10.1186/1472-6963-14-186

Chapter 7

# Adolescents Romantic Relationship: Dynamics of Parent-Child Relationship from India

*Navaneetham Janardhana and Basavaraj Manjula*


## Abstract

Increased interest in romantic relationships is central in adolescents' lives and has long been considered defining features of adolescence. Romantic relationships have significant influence on emotional wellbeing of adolescents. In Indian context, scientific literature on adolescent girls in romantic relationship is very minimal and studies focused upon sexuality-related issues and pre-marital sexual relationship. Due to social and cultural aspects, few adolescent girls who are involved in romantic relationship run away from home. These girls would come under care and protection under many circumstances such as child marriage, teenage pregnancy, sexual abuse, etc. The present study analyses the case reports in understanding the issues of adolescents in RR issues and the process of interventions provided. A total of 50 girls who were in RR were selected for the study Mean age is 16.34 years (SD ± 0.93) with a range of 14–18 years. About 78% were from lower socio economic status. It is important to understand their issues to provide psycho social intervention and facilitate healthy transition to adulthood. This has implication for designing intervention based on development perspective. Always adolescents in romantic relationship are under the conflict over prioritizing between their parents versus their romantic partner, when they forced to choose one.


**Keywords:** adolescence, adolescent romantic relationship, parents

## 1. Introduction

Adolescence is a crucial period for every individual with ample rapid physical, psychological and social changes [1–3]. In this critical transitional phase, boys and girls progress from same-sex to other-sex relationships, including involvement with romantic partners. Growing social expectations for dating behaviors, biological motivations, socio-emotional intelligence, and cognitive maturity during adolescence promotes young people to engage in romantic relationships [4, 5]. Most adolescents in their conversations discussed romantic relationships with no discomfort and reported to have significant preoccupation and rumination which further cause for strong emotions [6]. Many adolescents, particularly girls, whether single or in a relationship tend to spend more time discussing romantic relationships and pondering over past or future relationships [7]. Hence, romantic involvement during adolescence has received much attention.

India has one of the fastest growing youth populations in the world. The vast majority of adolescents, (children in the 10–19 age group) account for 22.8% of the population of India and girls below 19 years of age constitute one-fourth of India's fast growing population [8]. There are 1.5 million girls in India under the age of 15 already married. Of these, 20% or approximately 300,000 are mothers to at least one child. They are more prone to trafficking, HIV infection, and Substance abuse. Only 1% adolescents receive quality counseling, health and medical services [9]. Many of these issues addressed through various government programmes, policies and school health programme, and adolescent education programmes [10].

Increased interest in romantic relationships is central in adolescents' lives and has long been considered defining features of adolescence [1]. Romantic relationships have significant influence on emotional wellbeing of adolescents. In western context, romantic relationship has gained developmental significance and majority of adolescents involved in romantic relationship. In Indian context, scientific literature on Adolescent girls in romantic relationship is very minimal and studies focused upon sexuality related issues and pre-marital sexual relationship [11–13]. Due to social and cultural aspects, few adolescent girls who are involved in romantic relationship run away from home. These girls would come under care and protection under many circumstances such as child marriage, teenage pregnancy, sexual abuse, etc. it is important to understand their issues to provide psycho social intervention and facilitate healthy transition to adulthood [11–13].

Adolescence is a period of transition from childhood to adulthood, where adolescents try to establish a personal sense of individual identity and feelings of self-worth. During Adolescence there are certain important developmental tasks, such as, development of an identity; the transformation of family relationships; the development of close relationship with peers; the development of sexuality; scholastic achievement and career planning. Romantic experiences are believed to influence the course of a number of above mentioned developmental tasks [6]. Increased interest in romantic relationships is central in adolescents' lives and has long been considered defining features of adolescence [14]. Romantic relationship during adolescence follows a developmental course. Initial interactions typically occur in mixed boy-girl groups; then group dating begins, with several pairs engaging in some activity together [15]. Romantic relationships been defined as 'mutually acknowledged on-going voluntary interactions; in comparison to most other peer relationships, romantic ones typically have a distinctive intensity, which is usually marked by expressions of affection and current or anticipated sexual behavior, of course, some behaviors are simultaneously affectionate and sexual in nature [10].

Romantic relationship initially conceptualized as relatively unimportant compared to adults' relationships, adolescent romantic relationships have been shown in research to be often long term and bear significant resemblance to the features of adult romantic relationships [16, 17]. It is only within the last 2 decades that researchers have considered the potential impact of romantic experiences on adolescents' functioning. Since last 2 decades, academician and researchers have conducted research to understand romantic relationship among adolescents.

## 2. The understanding adolescent romantic relationship in the Indian context

Cultures vary widely in the norms, attitudes, and customs surrounding marriage. Marriage is a sacred institution in India [18], with long-established norms and customs with strict cultural sanctions against those who do not follow such unwritten norms [19]. In India unlike west, do not have a concept of 'dating'. The concept of dating is not heard by many adolescents, any attraction or liking of opposite sex ends up in marriage. Children are expected to be under the control and supervision of their parents until their marriage. Parents act as protector and also as provider for their children until they are married. When a boy and girl in romantic relationship would elope or runaway for getting married, mainly because of their parents not approving their relationship nor agreeing for their marriage. Caste, religion, socio economic status, character, etc., are important factors for marriage. In West, individuals select their own marital partner, whereas in India, parents and the extended family members select the marital partner and ensure that the partner is a good match within their caste and family network [20].

Janardhana et al., [21] in their reports of proving psycho social interventions for children in difficult circumstances under the care and protection of Child Welfare Committee (annual and six monthly reports) and in their studies Janardhana and Manjula [12, 13, 21] have mentioned about individual, family and other factors associated with romantic relationship. Adolescent girls in romantic relationship were aged between 13 and 18 years. Few were dropped out of school, majority of them are high school/college going. More than half of the adolescents in romantic relationship had poor academic performance and low academic achievement motivation. Few adolescents girls were asked to stop studies because parents knew about their romantic relationship. They had poor knowledge about personal safety, sexuality and reproductive health. Alcohol in parents, disturbed family routine, parental discord, poor parental supervision and monitoring, poor quality of relationship between parents and children, poor communication between parents and children, rejection of girls by their parents are some of the family factors associated with adolescent in romantic relationship. Caste, socio economic status, boy's background were some of the main reasons for their rejection of romantic relationship.

Perceptions and attitudes towards romantic relationships have evolved in the Indian context. In the current scenario, meeting socially for companionship and going beyond companionship has become quite popular among adolescents particularly those residing in urban areas. Dating was considered taboo decades ago, but now, it is quite common. Adolescent dating culture has been noted to be increasing in the country [22]. In India, globalization, urbanization, rapid economic growth and the extensive reach of media has changed the realities of young people in just a generation. Young people are exposed to new ideas and are better informed about their rights and responsibilities. The declining age of puberty and the increasing age of marriage have created a growing window of opportunities in which young people more chances to engage premarital romantic and sexual relationships [23].

## 3. Cultural context of marriage in India

India being a collectivist culture allows families to play a dominant role in taking major decisions centering lives of children and adolescents. Choice marriages are still discouraged and parental acceptance is crucial for marriage. Parents often believe that strict supervision of children inhibits their formation of romantic or sexual partnerships [24]. Despite strict supervision, disapproval of interactions with opposite gender, there are opportunities for social mixing and young people have devised ways of developing romantic partnerships with the opposite sex [25]. These emphases on how adolescents in India are fascinated between conflicting ideas. It has been observed that on one hand adolescents have strong desires for romantic exploration and on other hand strict parental supervision and traditional values on premarital relationships. This has led to the expansion of research interest in the area and has resulted in various research initiatives.

With changes from parent-arranged marriages to dating, individual choice courtship emerged as an activity in its own right, creating a new institution in culture. It involves individual choice with a defined time period. It also differs from parent-arranged marriages in the aspect of sexual permissiveness, the extent to which couples physically intimate before marriage [26].

The dimensions of individualism and collectivism are key constructs in understanding the social structuring of relationships. In individualistic societies like America, romantic love is an important base for marriage where love is known to promote personal growth through the relationship. Whereas, marriage in collectivistic societies such as India love and intimacy were less important factors, however, studies among young adults show signs of change towards greater valuing of love as a basis for marriage [27].

Regarding gender differences and choice marriage, the Indian woman's self-construct is more suggestive of a relational rather than individualized self. The joint family system structures the woman's relationships as well as prepares her to undertake the roles of a wife and mother. After marriage, the sources of emotional intimacy are the mother-child relationship and that with other women in the household [28].

The socialization process plays an important role in Indian context, as girls restricted to have interaction with opposite gender apart from apart from male members of her family. There was a common perception among parents to think of their daughter's marriage soon after they attain menarche. To prevent premarital sexual behaviors many parents go for an early marriage of their daughter. Religious beliefs also seem to have a significant impact on attitudes towards sexuality [29]. However, with the growing awareness on prohibition of child marriage, education for girls and socio-economic-political changes in India age of marriage is increasing [30, 31].

Adolescent sexuality is known to be influenced by the interaction of multiple factors such as bio-psycho-social, economical, political, cultural and legal factors [32]. The institution of marriage regulates sexual relations; hence premarital sex is discouraged and disapproved. Social and religious sanctions against premarital sex have traditionally been strong determinants to its practice [33]. With the advent of socioeconomic development, there has been significant influence on the sexual attitude of adolescents. Currently, it has become more open and independent from the traditional ties and cultural norms on sexual behaviors.

## 4. Child protection mechanism and adolescent girls

In India there are several legislations, schemes and policies for wellbeing of children. One among them is Juvenile Justice (Care and Protection) Act, 2000 for providing care and protection to children in difficult circumstances. Adolescent girls in romantic relationship faces care and protection issue under following circumstances- run away from home with their romantic partners, getting married below legal age, sexual abuse by romantic partners, teenage pregnancy, interpersonal issues with parents for being in romantic involvement, etc. During the process of care and protection, adolescent girls come under institutional care for temporary period of time, they do require psycho social care, family counseling and legal support. The current study would focus on this population.

The Juvenile Justice (care and protection of children) Act 2015 is tone of the primary laws for children in need of care and protection. This is designed for the care, protection, development and rehabilitation of neglected children and delinquent juveniles, as well as for the adjudication of and disposal of certain matters related to them. This law is child-friendly and provides for the proper care, protection and rehabilitation of children in need of care and protection. A clear distinction has been made in the law between the juvenile offender and the children in difficult circumstances. The other salient features of this enactment are: (i) it prescribes a uniform age of 18 years below which both boys and girls are to be treated as children (ii) the Act directs that the cases related to juveniles should be completed within a period of 4 months (iii) it has been made compulsory to set up a Juvenile Justice Board (previously known as Juvenile Court) and Child Welfare Committee either for a District or a group of Districts. (iv) Special emphasis has been given for rehabilitation and social reintegration of the children and the alternatives provided for this are adoption, foster care, sponsorship and after-care. The new Act allows for the adoption of a child within the purview of this Act by any community [34].

Integrated Child Protection Scheme (ICPS): The scheme is a central government sponsored mechanism that aims to introduce and implement an effective system of child protection that rests on the cardinal principles of "protection of child rights" and "best interest of the child". It seeks convergence of the governmental and non-governmental/civil society sectors for creation of a safety net for children through integration of various preventive, curative, rehabilitation and protection services. There are wide range of services for children to ensure care and protection of children. These include institutional and non-institutional care and services, child line, foster care, sponsorship, shelter homes, promotion of family based care, after care programmes, adoption, Health, education, vocational training, development programmes, legal assistance and rehabilitation, etc. These services have been delivered at the district level through District Child Protection unit and statutory bodies such as Child Welfare Committee and Juvenile Justice Boards have been actively involved in ensuring protection of children.

Adolescent mental health is an integral part of School mental health programmes focuses on developmental needs of children and adolescents and focusing on prevention of high risk behaviors and promotion of mental health among them [35]. School Mental Health Programmes in India focused upon Life Skills education, Developmental needs, substance use, Sexuality, HIV/AIDS, Mental Health Orientation to teachers, student enrichment, etc. Manuals were prepared as part of program [36].

Increased interest in romantic relationship is the central part of their life and considered as defining features of adolescence. Existing literature on Adolescent romantic relationship highlighted that, Romantic relationship becomes increasingly significant in the lives of young people as they move from early to late adolescence [37]. It is one among the important developmental tasks in adolescence [15] and can influence the course of other developmental tasks [38]. The quality of adolescent romantic relationships can have long lasting effects on self-esteem and shape personal values regarding romance, intimate relationships, and sexuality [39, 40]. While healthy romantic relationships have many potential benefits for youth, unhealthy relationships pose risks that may have long-lasting impact [41].

### 4.1 Methods

The present study aimed at understanding the psychosocial issues of adolescent girls in RR under care and protection framework. This study was carried out as part of a project providing psychosocial interventions for children in difficult circumstances under the care and protection of child welfare committee, supported by Karnataka state integrated child protection society, Government of Karnataka. The researchers are from the Department of Psychiatric Social Work, National Institute of Mental Health And Neuro Sciences, providing services for the children in difficult circumstances referred from child welfare committee on daily basis. Children, who are referred from the CWC for temporary institutional care in the children home, constitute same for the study. Children speaking Kannada, Telugu and English constitute the sample for the study. Children reporting to be above 18 years (with documentary proof were excluded from the study as they would not be governed by child welfare committee. Psychosocial care was provided to adolescent girls in RR, under care and protection issues. Case reports, with detail notes of the therapist was documented, the present study analyses the case reports in understanding the issues of adolescents in RR issues and the process of interventions provided. The individual files have been maintained by a psychiatric social worker, eliciting information about the RR, marriage with the romantic partner, reason for run away with the marital partner, and to their decisions about their future life, carrier and family life.

The cases seen in 8 months were taken for the study. Ethical aspects were taken into consideration with regard to maintaining anonymity of the participants; the study findings does not affect the dignity of children, and they all received psychosocial care services as part of the project. Initially, frequency analysis was done with regard to socio demographic variables, themes were identified and later codes were made to understand the individual and family issues related to adolescents in RR. The data was analyzed using R software, and frequency analysis was done.

### 4.2 Results

Fifty girls who were in RR were selected for the study Mean age is 16.34 years (SD ± 0.93) with a range of 14–18 years. About 60% were in high school, 32% of them were in Pre University College. One joined for BE (bachelor of engineering) and remaining did not attend formal education. About 50% of the participants discontinued their studies, 20% of them completed the course, 14% were currently pursuing the course and 10% had dropped from studies. About 78% were from lower socio economic status, 18% from middle socio economic status and 4% from higher socio economic status. About 80% belonged to Hindu religion, 12% belonged to Christian religion, and remaining 8% belonged to Muslim religion. The mean age of menarche is 12.46. About 56% of the participants are from nuclear family, 26% from single parent families and remaining 18% are from joint family (**Table 1**).

Little more than 95% of the adolescent girls in RR ran away with their romantic partner. Remaining 6% of participants did not run away from home; however they came under care and protection mechanisms on the request of parents. The reason for run away with their romantic partner was to get married (62%) and another 38% of them had ambiguity regarding their marriage with the romantic partner. Little more than 70% of the adolescent girls believed that having sexual intercourse with their romantic partner would get their marriage approval. Most Adolescents reported that marriage gave them sanction for the sexual relationship. Another 28% of them did not have sexual relationship. Nearly 76% were not aware about the safe sex practices, sexual health, reproductive health, and pregnancy, etc. (**Table 2**).

The case files analysis reveals that most adolescents were worried about parent's rejection of their romantic partner and had guilt feeling that they were not able to

| Sl. No. | Variable | Frequency N = 50 | Percentage |
|---|---|---|---|
| 1 | Age | Mean 16.34 SD ± 0.939 | |
| 2 | Education | High school 30<br>Pursuing PUC 16<br>No formal education 03<br>Pursuing BE 01 | 60%<br>32% |
| 3 | Status of education | Completed 10<br>Discontinued 25<br>Drop out 5<br>No formal education 3<br>Ongoing 7 | 20%<br>50%<br>10%<br>06%<br>14% |
| 4 | Socio economic status | High 2<br>Middle 9<br>Low 39 | 4%<br>18%<br>78% |
| 5 | Religion | Hindu 40<br>Muslim 4<br>Christian 6 | 80%<br>8%<br>12% |
| 6 | Age at menarche | Mean 12.46 | |
| 7 | Type of family | Joint 9<br>Nuclear 28<br>Single parent 13 | 18%<br>56%<br>26% |

**Table 1.**
*Personal profile of the adolescents in romantic relationship.*

meet the expectations of parents nor they were able to fulfill the dreams of their parents. Most adolescents were also aware that their romantic involvement has been one of the reasons for academic decline; some have to be dropped out from schools as their parents knew about their romantic relationships. Parents started restricting their movement by stopping to attend school. Always adolescents in romantic relationship are under the conflict over prioritizing between their parents vs. their romantic partner, when they forced to choose one.

Adolescents in romantic relationship are also worried about legal action against their romantic partner, they wanted their romantic partners to be out from the correctional settings, and they do not want their romantic partner to be punished alone. Often Adolescents in romantic relationship are confused about prioritizing between going back to their family or to go back with their romantic partner. Adolescents feel that they have brought dishonor to the family. They are more worried about the reactions of their family members, especially extended relatives and neighbors. This confusion would govern their decision making about going to back along with their parents or to be in the rehabilitation center, wait for their romantic partners. They would be confused to take decisions about child bearing issues, as they are under aged and physically weak to bear the child in their womb.

Disturbed family functioning due to conflict over daughter's relationship, challenges in dealing with behavioral issues of adolescents in romantic relationship context, parenting issues like balancing warmth and control, accepting adolescent's autonomy, and deviance behavior. Parents finds difficult to accept daughter's decision about their romantic partner, and would be in a helpless situation of not able to convince their daughter about their reason of caste and the economic conditions for rejecting their selection. Social issues such as family honor, parents find it difficult to explain and answer to their relatives and neighbors. Parents find difficult

| At individual level | At family level |
|---|---|
| **Psychosocial issues identified before coming under care and protection** | |
| 1. Disturbed relationship with parents, and siblings at home due to romantic involvement<br>2. Problems in prioritizing their tasks and responsibilities<br>3. Lack of adequate knowledge regarding sexuality and reproductive health and personal safety skills<br>4. Lack of skills in analyzing the situation and decision making regarding academics, marriage and sexual activities with romantic partner<br>5. Lack of skills in foreseeing the consequences of run away from home with the romantic partner | 1. Disagreement regarding the selection of romantic partner because of caste, family status of the boy, physical appearance, the character of the boy and family honor.<br>2. Parents become critical and punitive<br>3. The disturbed parent-child relationship in the process of discussion about marriage with the romantic partner<br>4. Parents made efforts to prevent their daughter to dissolve their romantic relationship in the form of<br>5. Forceful marriage attempt to prevent their daughter to get married to her romantic partner<br>6. Restriction of activities in the form of not sending her outside, restriction of movement at home, no access to phone/mobile phone, not allowing them to meet friends, etc. to prevent them from involving in activities with romantic partner<br>7. Restriction to attend school/college and not supporting for continuing education because of fear of runaway behavior and meeting of romantic partner |
| **Psychosocial issues identified after coming under care and protection** | |
| 1. Lack of understanding about care and protection mechanism when they were brought to child welfare committee and placed in children homes.<br>2. Fear of legal action on the romantic partner because of runaway, sexual contact and marriage<br>3. Fear of parental reaction for their behavior<br>4. Fear of facing parents and inhibition to respond to their questions and discuss with them<br>5. Fear of rejection from parents for reintegration with family<br>6. Fear of lack of support from parents for continuing studies<br>7. Fear of not being able to get married to the romantic partner and forceful marriage with someone else after reintegrating with family<br>8. Fear of response from relatives, friends and neighbors after reintegrating with family<br>9. In case of pregnancy dilemma regarding childbearing versus termination of pregnancy<br>10. The dilemma in prioritizing romantic partner and parents in case of rigidity from parents | 1. Disturbed family functioning<br>2. Social, emotional and economic impact on family following the incident in the form of criticism and comments from relatives, neighbors, school, spending money in the process of tracing girl, accompanying to the hospital, court, legal procedures, dealing with their emotions regarding daughter, family honor<br>3. Social factors versus daughter's needs—Prioritizing are the major challenges for parents. As romantic relationship during adolescence has not received social acceptance, parents who are bound with social norms and social pressure face difficulties in accepting their daughter.<br>4. The dilemma in consenting for reintegration with family due to fear of the reoccurrence of behaviors in the romantic relationship context<br>5. Challenges in parenting adolescents with behavioral issues in the romantic relationship context |

**Table 2.**
*Provides information about the psychosocial issues among adolescents and their families.*

to cope with issues like, first time entering into the police station for registering complaint and attending judicial court procedures. Parents are often confused in prioritizing between importance of Social factors versus understanding daughter's decision and needs.

Based on the above understanding the authors are proposing a conceptual understanding of romantic relationship in the Indian context.

**Figures 1** and **2** describe the psychosocial issues identified among adolescents girls and their families. These model (as the figure is given below this text).

The above model depicts several factors associated with romantic involvement of adolescent girls. Modeling and learning from others' experiences play an important role in developing perceptions of romantic involvement and concept of ideal partner and ideal relationships. Understanding on healthy and unhealthy relationships in romantic involvement also one of the determinant of forming romantic relationship. This enables them to have norms in their relationship and to prepare for engage in healthy relationships.

The socialization process, socio-cultural norms on marriage, premarital relationships add to their concept of ideal romantic relationships and frames expectations on romantic partner. These influence them to look for stable relationships. Adolescents from late adolescence, school going with average academic performance had shown interest in forming romantic relationship. Adolescents hailing from lower socioeconomic status and difficult family situations, changes in family structure followed by transition such as single parent family, living with extended family members have higher chances of engage in romantic involvement. Poor parental monitoring and supervision of activities of adolescent girls may leave the unattended, which may impact on parent-adolescent relationship in future.

Romantic partner's characteristics are major determinants of forming romantic relationship and the quality of relationship between romantic partners. Adolescent girls formed romantic relationship with young/middle adults, who belonged to lower socioeconomic status and hailed from different caste. The

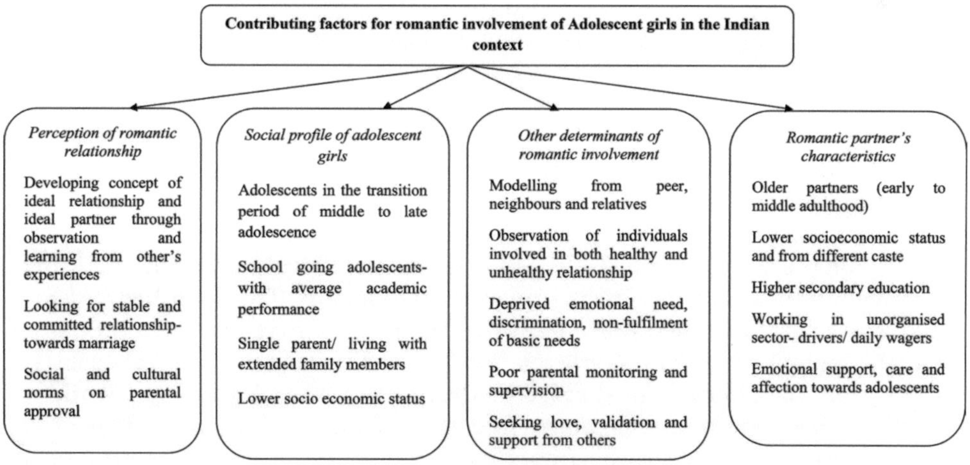


**Figure 1.**
*Factors contributing for romantic relationship in the Indian context. Note: Conceptual frame work was written based on the on the observations from the project of Dr. N Janardhana, Principal Investigator, 'psychosocial interventions for children in difficult circumstances', supported by KSICPS, Government of Karnataka and the doctoral research of MS Manjula, guided by Dr. N. Janardhana and Dr. Nirmala B.P.*

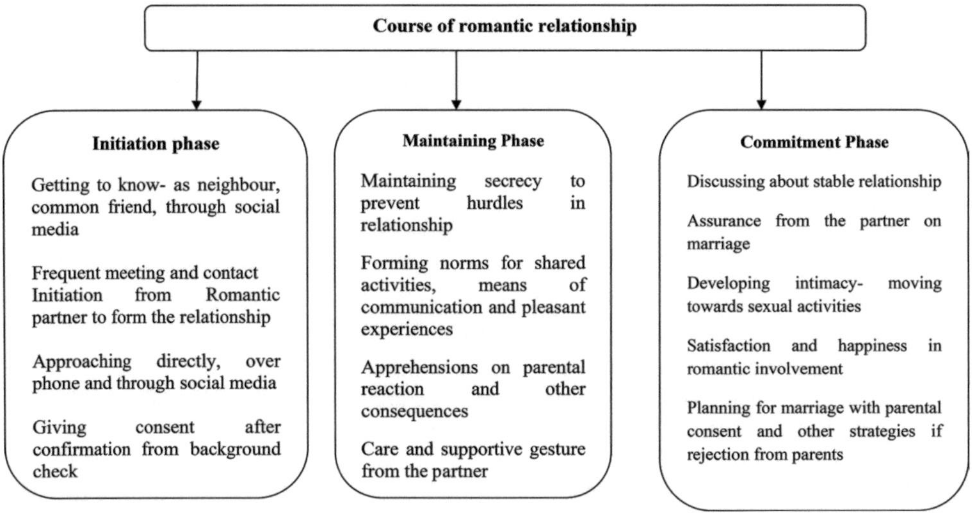


**Figure 2.**
*The course of romantic relationship. Note: Conceptual frame work for understanding the course of romantic relationship was written based on the on the observations from the project of Dr. N Janardhana, Principal Investigator, 'psychosocial interventions for children in difficult circumstances', supported by KSICPS, Government of Karnataka and the doctoral research of MS Manjula, guided by Dr. N. Janardhana and Dr. Nirmala B.P.*

deprived emotional needs were fulfilled by their romantic partners and their needs were acknowledged and validated. Romantic partners were source of support and encouragement and they felt happy in their presence and contributed for quality of relationship.

The course of romantic relationship is been given in the below diagram based on initiation phase, middle phase and commitment phase. The process of romantic relationship been described based on the experiences of adolescents in romantic relationship. Relationship in the below diagram described how the friendship got turned into infatuation and then eloping with their boyfriend to get marriage so that their marriage gets recognized from their parents (**Figure 2**).

## 5. Psychosocial interventions for adolescent girls and their families in romantic relationship context

Based on the above understanding of romantic relationship, we have delivered following interventions for girls in romantic relationship[1]. The described psychosocial issues provided the framework for developing the psychosocial intervention for adolescent girls in the romantic relationship and their families. Psychosocial interventions have been formed based on the Social casework and group work approach. These interventions categorized as individual interventions, family interventions (sessions with parents and conjoint sessions with parents and adolescent).

[1] Conceptual frame work for understanding the course of romantic relationship was written based on the on the observations from the project of Dr N Janardhana, Principal Investigator, 'psychosocial interventions for children in difficult circumstances', supported by KSICPS, Government of Karnataka and the doctoral research of MS Manjula, guided by Dr N. Janardhana and Dr Nirmala B. P.

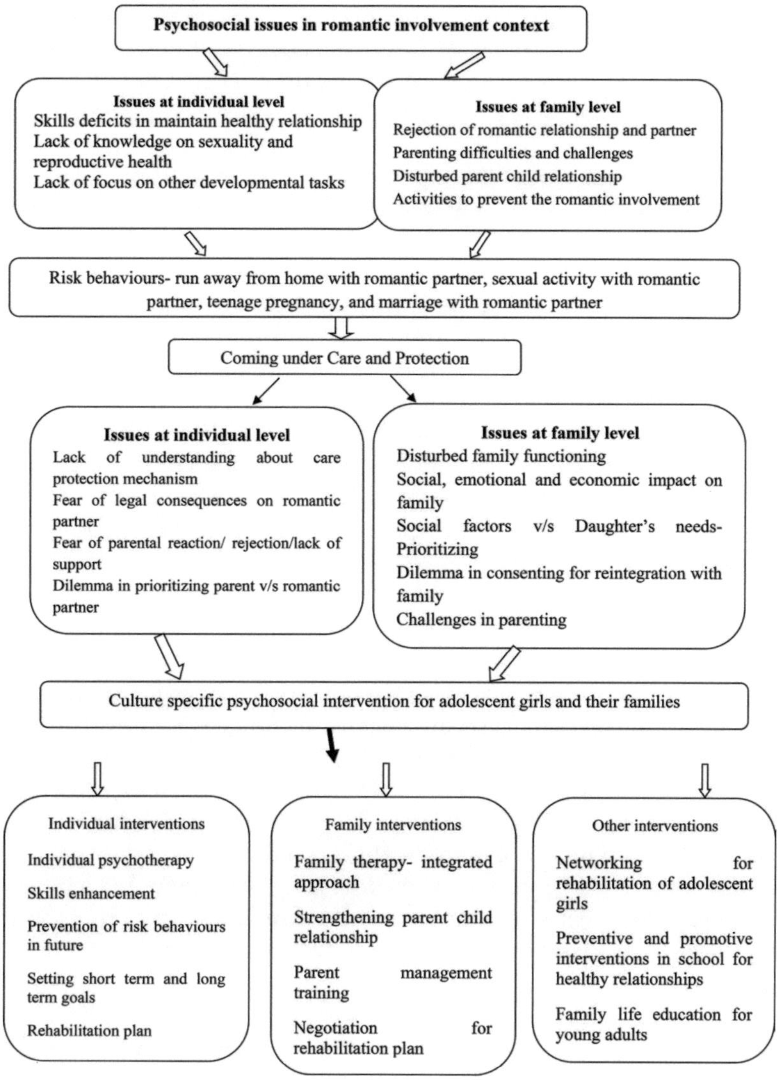


## 6. Psychosocial interventions

Individual interventions with adolescent girls aimed at enhancing psychosocial competence among adolescent girls to deal effectively with the psychosocial issues and facilitate them fulfill the developmental tasks of adolescence. To achieve this aim, preventive, promotive, curative and rehabilitative approaches can be adopted.

## 7. Psycho social intervention for families of adolescent girls in romantic relationship

Working with family is an integral part for providing psycho-social interventions to adolescents. Family factors such as relationship with family members, early experiences in childhood, parenting practices, family dynamics, and parental response towards romantic involvement have contributed to partner selection and adopting risk behaviors among adolescents. Hence, it would be beneficial to give family interventions to this particular cohort. Family plays an important role in the process of care plan for adolescent girls and ensuring care and protection for them in the future. It is also essential to discuss the concerns of parents as romantic involvement of their daughter and associated issues can have significant impact on the family.

Family interventions emphasize upon systemic approach and different schools of family therapies are psycho-dynamic approach, structural family therapy, strategic family therapy, solution focused, problem solving, cognitive behavioral family therapy, psycho-education, narrative approach, integrated approach, etc.

The major issues identified at the family level are authoritative and punitive parenting, enmeshed boundaries, parental autonomy on children's marriage, impaired parent- child relationship, loss of trust and maladaptive coping strategies, etc. Families belong to the developmental life cycle stage of families with adolescent children reported significant challenges. For those families with dysfunctions, may need therapy sessions as either joint or conjoint sessions. The main aim of family interventions is to reduce risk factors in family, promote protective factors and enhance parent's skills to deal with the issues and safeguard care and protection of adolescents.

### 7.1 Curative approach

This approach focuses on providing therapeutic services for adolescent girls in the institutions and in a clinical setup. Specific techniques derived from different therapies such as Supportive psychotherapy, cognitive behavior therapy, Emotions focused therapy, Interpersonal relationship therapy, Solution focused therapy, Strength-based approach, Dialectical behavior therapy and Motivation enhancement therapy, etc. can be adopted in the therapy process.

Individual therapy sessions focus on addressing their thoughts, emotions and behaviors associated with romantic involvement and enhancing their abilities to deal with the current situations and crisis. Individual therapy can focus on the following areas.

- Establishing therapeutic alliance by being nonjudgmental, ensuring confidentiality, and emphasizing on their active participation in the therapy process.

- Supportive interventions using ventilation, emotional catharsis, validation of their concerns and experiences.

- Provide *education* on child protection mechanism, functions of Child Welfare Committee, activities in children home for girls, child protection personnel, the process of making care plan and services available for children and adolescents to ensure their safety and overall development.

- Insight facilitation: reflection on their perspectives on romantic involvement, process of selecting partner, commitment for stable relationship, their role in each phase of romantic involvement, decision making process in run away, sexual activity, marriage, pregnancy and childbearing, consequences of risk behaviors on different areas such as family, academics, mental health, social consequences and facilitating understanding on current situation from multiple perspectives.

- Adopting *cognitive approaches*: assessment of thought process on romantic involvement, sexuality and reproductive health, family life, academics and career goals and future plans; identifying and assessing cognitive errors, dysfunctional thinking negative automatic thoughts contributed for the current situation and future care plan is very essential. Cognitive strategies such as cognitive restructuring, development of alternative thinking, challenging dysfunctional thinking, distraction techniques can be used in the process.

- *Coping with emotion*: most of the adolescents experience humiliation, guilt, self-stigma, hopelessness, worthlessness. Enable them to be aware of their emotions, labeling their emotions, enhancing their abilities to express their emotions in a better way and regulation of emotions.

- *Behavioral interventions:* behavioral assessment of desired and undesired behaviors, risk behaviors, discussing on rewards for complying with desired behaviors, consequences of risk behaviors. Relaxation strategies can also be taught to relieve their anxiety.

- *Sexuality and reproductive health education*: addressing myths and misconceptions, attitude towards sexuality, social and cultural factors, decision-making process while consenting for sexual activities, consequences of risky sexual behaviors, safe sex practices, their perspective on teenage pregnancy and childbearing, pros and cons of childbearing and surrendering of a baby.

- *Setting short term and long term goals*: (depends on the age of the girl, goals to accomplish, for example, 3 months for next 3 years). Future orientation perspective and motivational interviewing technique can be used to facilitate girl to identify her interest in academics and career building, priorities in life. The goals may be completing education/training, rebuilding the trust of parents, seeking the job and becoming independent, getting married, etc.

- *Preparing for family sessions:* enabling adolescents to deal with their emotions (fear, anger, hostility) and negative thoughts which make them avoid to face their parents and other family members.

- *Problem-solving skills*: enable them to generate alternatives for care, evaluating pros and cons of each alternative, such as vocational training with placement and reintegration with home and studies/vocational training.

### 7.2 Promotive approach

The promotive approach focuses on the enhancement of skills and competence among adolescents. Following areas can be focused on the promotion of mental health among adolescent girls.

- *Skills enhancement*: life skills based activities to enable their skills on the healthy relationship in romantic involvement, setting boundaries, mutual respect, quality time, shared activities, norms in relationship.

- *Personal safety skills*: protecting from abuse in the relationship context, identifying risks for abuse and taking precautions, reporting and seeking help.

- *Legal awareness* on POCSO Act, prohibition of child marriage Act and legal implications of their risk-taking behavior.

- *Developmental education* to focus on developmental tasks during adolescence need for fulfilling other tasks such as academics, career, family relationships, sexuality and peer relationship along with the romantic relationship.

Identifying their needs, challenges and support required to meet these developmental tasks and facilitating the same.

### 7.3 Preventive approach

- Prevention of further risk behaviors in future—facilitate discussion with the girl on identifying triggers/precipitating factors which may make them repeat risk-taking behaviors and enable their critical thinking to come up with strategies to address them.
- Preparing them Emphasize upon healthy relationship during courtship, adhere to law and advantages of following desired behaviors.
- Providing information on resource agencies and contact details to seek help during the crisis.
- Enable them to face the social consequences such as criticism, labeling and cope effectively.

## 8. Psychosocial intervention for families of adolescent girls in the romantic relationship

Working with family is an integral part of providing Psycho-Social interventions for adolescents. Family factors such as the relationship with family members, early experiences in family, parenting practices, family dynamics, and parental response towards romantic involvement have contributed to romantic involvement and risk behaviors among adolescents. Hence, it is very important to have family interventions. Apart from these, family plays a crucial role in the process of care plan for adolescent girls and ensuring care and protection in the future. It is also essential to address their concerns too as a romantic involvement of their daughter and associated issues have a significant impact on the family.

Family interventions emphasize upon systemic approach and family therapy services can be formed based on different schools of family therapy such as structural family therapy, strategic family therapy, solution focused, problem-solving, cognitive behavioral family therapy, integrated approach, etc.

The major issues identified at the family level are authoritative and punitive parenting, enmeshed boundaries, parental autonomy on children's marriage, impaired parent-adolescent relationship, loss of trust and maladaptive coping strategies, etc. These families are in the family life stage of families with adolescents and reported significant challenges. Family therapy sessions can be carried out as joint and conjoint sessions. The main aim of family interventions is to prevent risk factors in the family, promote protective factors and enhance parent's skills to deal with the issues and ensure care and protection of adolescents.

Individual sessions with parents or conjoint parent-adolescent can focus on the following areas in the family interventions;

1. *Supportive interventions*: facilitating ventilation and validation of their concerns and seeking their active participation in the therapy and care plan process. It also looks in to the coping strategies of parents and designed to treat parent behavior, parent mental health, adolescent behavior, family function, etc.

2. *Emotion focused therapy*: parents perceive romantic involvement of their adolescent daughter as shameful act and express anger/hostility towards them.

Parental distress could be due to diminishing family's honor, legal procedures, social and economic consequences because of runaway behavior. Hence, addressing their emotions is very essential. Emotion focused therapy help them to deal with the emotions and prevents their behaviors/decisions driven by their emotions. Facilitating forgiveness and building trust between parent and adolescent is very essential in the process of rebuilding their relationship and care plan for ensuring care and protection of adolescents.

3. *Insight facilitation*: It includes reflective exercises on family factors such as quality of relationship among family members, parenting style, decision-making in the family, general family emotional environment, communication patterns, family values and attitudes, etc. These above-mentioned factors can act as precipitating or contributing for romantic involvement and risk behaviors among adolescents. This particular approach would help parents to understand, acknowledge and bring changes behavior and the way they deal with daughter's romantic involvement.

4. *Psycho-education*: It acknowledges parents perspectives and beliefs, socio-cultural influence on adolescent romantic relationship and their disapproval of romantic involvement of daughter. At the same time bringing attitudinal changes by giving developmental perspective and other factors associated with romantic involvement. This approach emphasizes on romantic involvement as normative process and how it affects adolescents.

5. *Parent management skills*: It helps in altering faulty parenting styles while dealing with adolescent issues and enhances open communication (negotiation, expressing concerns). It boosts mutual norms and healthy parenting to address temperament or behavioral issues. Role play method could use to enhance their skills, prescriptive parenting—clarifying dos and don'ts for next 2 years.

- *Family life cycle stages-challenges and role of parents*: educating parents about family life cycle stages-especially on families with adolescents, about challenges and tasks. Emphasis is on role of parents in education, training, facilitating healthy transition to adulthood. As most of the adolescents moved to the next stage, it is essential to discuss about marriage and decision-making process.

- *Ensuring family support for adolescent to fulfill responsibilities*: discuss about their support for facing challenges in community and responding to criticism, supporting each other, etc., which would help girl to focus on other developmental tasks such as education, career planning, healthy peer and family relationships.

Conjoint sessions with parents and adolescent girls can focus on the following areas:

- *Strengthening quality of parent and adolescent relationship* through rebuilding trust and family bond, facilitating mutual validation of their concerns, emphasize on significance of quality of relationship and its influence on bringing desired behavioral and attitudinal changes.

- *Communication skills:* focusing on opportunity for open and direct communication and addressing barriers for expressiveness in the family, active listening, acknowledging concerns, clear communication and seeking clarifications on meaning, and intentions. Encouraging negotiation between parent and adolescent and emphasize on consensus on the accepted behaviors and mutual expectations.

- *Structural changes*: here focus is on healthy boundaries between adolescent and parents, setting clear boundaries on areas of parental involvement. Here it is very essential to discuss autonomy of adolescents and role of parents, at the same time ensuring autonomy of parent to prevent risky behaviors.

- *Problem solving approach*: here emphasis is on address their concerns on supporting girl's education/vocational training, reintegration with family. Ensure active participation of both adolescent girl and parents in generating healthy alternatives. Facilitate seeking clarification, sharing mutual concerns and reaching consensus about studies, reintegration with family or placement in organizations.

- *Behavioral approach*: discusses on expectations, setting norms for dos and don'ts in conjoint sessions. Facilitating both adolescent girl and parents discuss on their expectations from each other, reaching consensus on expected behaviors and non-acceptable behaviors. They can also negotiate for rewards for desired behaviors and consequences of undesired behaviors.

## 9. Discussion

The course of the romantic relationship identified knowledge about romantic partner, strategies used by romantic partner or respondents to initiate the relationship, process of accepting and forming the relationship, discussing about maintaining relationship—open versus hiding relationship, factors contributed them to take decision of run away from home, their quality of relationship and intimacy.

In the current study, romantic partner were first met in the neighborhood, near the area of residence or school, on the way to school or through social media. Most of them were familiar to each other and thus initiated the friendship. In most of the cases, boys took the initiative to propose by approaching directly, through common friends, telephonic conversations or through social media like Facebook. It is interesting to note that men initiated the relationship forming, which shows the socio-culture influence in initiating the relationship. Though respondents had more expressiveness, with regard to initiating the relationship they were shy, had inhibitions. Hence, they have taken time to respond to agree to the relationship. Meantime they focused on background check with close friends and get convinced before saying yes for the relationship. However, most of them were not completely aware about the family background of the romantic partners. During the course of the relationship, they tried to maintain the secrecy from family and peers to avoid the complications. Most of them thought of getting married after few years with the consent of parents.

Studies on premarital relationships among youth in India demonstrated that despite strict parental supervision, girls found ways of forming romantic friendships and engaging in sexual relations [41]. During the later stages of the relationship, when the family got to know about their romantic involvement, they had decided to elope with their romantic partner due to fear of family, lack parental approval and punitive behaviors to prevent their romantic involvement. Similar results were found in the case reports and quantitative results. Run away from home was used as the immediate solution to continue in romantic involvement and avoid issues in the family. In a study on dynamics of parent-child relationship in romantic involvement context, lack of parental support for choice marriage, restrictive parenting style were found as major issues [12].

The days spend with romantic partner developed intimacy—initially as a force from romantic partner and also for the social reasons like sex as a means to convince family for the marriage and current marital status as an approval to engage in physical intimacy. Studies on sexuality and reproductive health behaviors among youths in India identified physical intimacy among youth both in romantic and non-romantic context, safe and unsafe sexual behaviors [42–44]. While staying with their romantic partner they received care, supportive gesture and open communication, which indicates the quality of relationship with their romantic partner and they were the main source of emotional support to them.

The above findings on course on romantic relationship are similar to the romantic involvement model during adolescence; Initiation Phase—beginning of interest in the opposite sex; superficial selection process; interactions are weak attempts at establishing a romantic relationship (physical characteristics); Affiliation Phase—observes behaviors and attitudes; focus on companionship (social characteristics); Intimate Phase—focus of the paired relationship is intimacy (deep feelings of emotional attachment) and often sexual activity and the last phase; Committed Phase—adolescent romantic relationships are established and exclusive at times, resembling the marriage relationship; more intense relationships; more caring towards their romantic partner; better at resolving conflict within the relationship [45].

Interventions for adolescents to deal with their RR includes rapport establishment, not taking sides of either adolescent or their parents. Interventions started with their understanding of personal safety, sexuality and reproductive health, and its importance. Discussions were held on the legal framework governing children in India. Help adolescent to look at their developmental tasks like academic involvement or vocational training. Support was extended to adolescents to set short term and long term goals. Preventive and promotive mental health interventions for enhancing psychosocial competence were provided. Supportive therapeutic interventions could assist adolescent girls to learn healthy ways of relating to others [46]. Helping professionals need to recognize, respond to the issues and problems of adolescent in RR [47]; dealing with their relationship with the parents; dealing with the community attitudes; building support network. Carlson [48] asserted that counselors working with youth must not only recognize violent actions, but also seek to understand the underlying issues causing such behavior.

Under the project entitled "psychosocial interventions for children in difficult circumstances" services were provided at the children home for girls, Bangalore. Adolescent girls and their families those who approached Child Welfare Committee in romantic involvement context were also received psychosocial interventions. The above mentioned areas of interventions were provided to them based on their needs and issues and found to be useful in this set up [12, 13, 48].

## 10. Conclusion

Romantic relationship during adolescence has received developmental significance and has both positive and negative outcomes for adolescents. Many adolescents due to many factors like high risk behaviors, unhealthy relationship, violation of legal norms and others force them to be in crisis situation. This affects their relationship with family, academics and other opportunities, affecting their development process. Providing interventions to these children and adolescents is important. Understanding adolescent issues from developmental perspective helps in designing programmes for adolescents and their family members. This would facilitate healthy transition to adulthood and enables them to take part in societal development.

## Author details

Navaneetham Janardhana[1*] and Basavaraj Manjula[2]

1 Department of Psychiatric Social Work, NIMHANS, Bangalore, India

2 Narayana Hrudayalaya, Bangalore, India

*Address all correspondence to: janardhannimhans@gmail.com

## References

[1] Blakemore SJ, Burnett S, Dahl RE. The role of puberty in the developing adolescent brain. Human Brain Mapping. 2010;**31**(6):926-933

[2] Christie D, Viner R. ABC of adolescence: Adolescent development. British Medical Journal. 2005;**330**(7486):301

[3] Rice FP, Dolgin KG. The Adolescent: Development, Relationships and Culture. New Zealand: Pearson Education; 2005

[4] Connolly J, Craig W, Goldberg A, Pepler D. Conceptions of cross-sex friendships and romantic relationships in early adolescence. Journal of Youth and Adolescence. 1999;**28**(4):481-494

[5] Furman W. Friends and lovers: The role of peer relationships in adolescent romantic relationships. In: Relationships as Developmental Contexts. United Kingdom: Psychology Press; 1999. pp. 147-168

[6] Furman W, ShaVer L. The Role of Romantic Relationships in Adolescent Development: Wyndol Furman and Laura Shaffer. InAdolescent romantic relations and sexual behavior. Psychology Press; 18 Jul 2003. pp. 17-36

[7] Eder D. "Go get ya a French!": Romantic and sexual teasing among adolescent girls. Paper presented at the An earlier version of this chapter was presented at a conference on Gender Roles Through the Life Span at Ball State U, Muncie, IN. 1993

[8] Sciences, I. I. f. P., & International, M. National Family Health Survey (NFHS-3), 2005-06. India: IIPS Mumbai; 2007

[9] Mission NH. Adolescent Health. National Health Mission Components: RMNCH+A: Adolescent Health India: Government of India. 2013. Available from: http://nrhm.gov.in/nrhm-components/rmnch-a/adolescent-health/adolescent-health/background.html

[10] Sivagurunathan C, Umadevi R, Rama R, Gopalakrishnan S. Adolescent health: Present status and its related programmes in India. Are we in the right direction? Journal of Clinical and Diagnostic Research: JCDR. 2015;**9**(3):LE01

[11] Janardhana N, Manjula B, Nirmala BP, Reddy K, Sagar JV, Roopesh BN. Psycho Social Intervention for Children in Difficult Circumstances. Quarterly report. Department of Women and Child Development, Karnataka, 2014, 2015. 2016

[12] Janardhana N, Manjula B. Infatuation and love of an adolescent girl: Dynamics of parent child relationship. Indian Journal of Child Health. 2018;**5**(2):99-103

[13] Janardhana N, Manjula B. Psycho social intervention for adolescents in relationship issues under the care and protection of child welfare committee. Journal of Indian Association for Child & Adolescent Mental Health. 2018;**14**(1):40-59

[14] Sullivan HS. The Interpersonal Theory of Psychiatry. New York: Norton; 1953

[15] Connolly J, Craig W, Goldberg A, Pepler D. Mixed-gender groups, dating, and romantic relationships in early adolescence. Journal of Research on Adolescence. 2004;**14**(2):185-207

[16] Collins WA. More than myth: The developmental significance of romantic relationships during adolescence. Journal of Research on Adolescence. 2003;**13**(1):1-24

[17] Larson RW et al. The emotions of romantic relationships: Do they wreak havoc on adolescents? In: Furman W, Brown BB, Feiring C, editors. The Development of Romantic Relationships in Adolescence. Cambridge: Cambridge University Press; 1999. pp. 19-49

[18] Marshall TC. Cultural differences in intimacy: The influence of gender-role ideology and individualism-collectivism. Journal of Social and Personal Relationships. 2008;**25**:43-168

[19] Netting N. Marital ideoscapes in 21st century India: Creative combination of love and responsibility. Journal of Family Issues. 2010;**31**:707-726

[20] Myers JE, Madathil J, Tingle LR. Marriage satisfaction and wellness in India and the United States: A preliminary comparison of arranged marriages and marriages of choice. Journal of Counseling & Development. 2005;**83**:183-190

[21] Janardhana N, Manjula B. Adolescent girls in care and protection framework for their romantic relationship. Institutionalised Children Explorations and Beyond. 2017;**4**(1):24-31

[22] Varma P, Mathur A. Adolescent romantic relationships. The International Journal of Indian Psychology. 2015;**3**(1):15-27

[23] Alexander M, Garda L, Kanade S, Jejeebhoy S, Ganatra B. Correlates of premarital relationships among unmarried youth in Pune district, Maharashtra, India. International Family Planning Perspectives. 1 Dec 2007:150-159

[24] Sodhi G, Verma M, Pelto PJ. Seeking gratification: A study of sexual behaviour patterns of adolescents in an urban slum. Reproductive Health in India: New Evidence. Jaipur, India: Rawat Publications; 2008. pp. 303-322

[25] Mehra S, Savithri R, Coutinho L. Sexual behaviour among unmarried adolescents in Delhi, India: Opportunities despite parental controls. In: Paper presented at the IUSSP Regional Population Conference, Bangkok, June. 2002

[26] Olsen D, DeFrain J. Marriage and the Family: Diversity and Strengths. Mountain View, CA: Sage; 1994

[27] Dion KK, Dion KL. Individualistic and collectivistic perspectives on gender and the cultural context of love and intimacy. Journal of Social Issues. 1993;**49**(3):53-69

[28] Kumar U. Life stages in the development of the Hindu woman in India. In: Women in Crosscultural Perspective. New York: Praeger; 1991

[29] Rangaiyan G. Sexuality and Sexual Behaviour in the Age of AIDS: A Study among College Youth in Mumbai. Mumbai, India: International Institute for Population Sciences; 1996

[30] Ghule M, Balaiah D, Joshi B. Attitude towards premarital sex among rural college youth in Maharashtra, India. Sexuality & Culture. 2007;**11**(4):1-17

[31] GOI. The Protection of Children from Sexual Offenses Act. New Delhi, India: The Gazette of india; 2012. Available from: http://wcd.nic.in/sites/default/files/childprotection31072012.pdf

[32] Bearinger LH, Sieving RE, Ferguson J, Sharma V. Global perspectives on the sexual and reproductive health of adolescents: Patterns, prevention, and potential. The Lancet. 2007;**369**(9568):1220-1231

[33] Christopher FS, Sprecher S. Sexuality in marriage, dating, and other relationships: A decade review. Journal of Marriage and Family. 2000;**62**(4):999-1017

[34] GOI. The Juvenile Justice (Care and Protection of Children) Act 2015. New Delhi India: The Gazet of India; 2016. Available from: http://cara.nic.in/PDF/JJ%20act%202015.pdf

[35] Bharath S, Kumar K V. The Activity Manual for Teachers on Health Promotion Using Life Skill Approach for 10th Standard. Bangalore: Department of Psychiatry, NIMHANS Publication; 2005

[36] Bharath S, Kumar KV, Mukesh YP. Clinical practice guidelines for school mental health program. Indian Journal of Psychiatry, CPG. 2008:307-321

[37] Chandrashekar CR. Manual on Students' Counselling for College Students. NIMHANS Publication; 2007

[38] Deanna Trella. Adolescents and romantic relationship education programs. NCFMR Research Brief 09-02. 2009

[39] Foshee VA, Bauman KE, Arriaga XB, Helms RW, Koch GG, Linder GF. An evaluation of safe dates, an adolescent dating violence prevention program. American Journal of Public Health. 1998;**88**(1):45-50

[40] Foshee VA, Foshee VA, Benefield T, Suchindran C, Ennett ST, Bauman KE, et al. The development of four types of adolescent dating abuse and selected demographic correlates. Journal of Research on Adolescence. 2009;**19**:380-400

[41] Furman W. The emerging field of adolescent romantic relationships. Current Directions in Psychological Science. 2002;**11**:177-180. DOI: 10.1111/1467-8721.00195

[42] Abraham L. Bhai-behen, true love, time pass: Friendships and sexual partnerships among youth in an Indian metropolis. Culture, Health & Sexuality. 2002;**4**(3):337-353

[43] Abraham L, Kumar KA. Sexual experiences and their correlates among college students in Mumbai City, India. International Family Planning Perspectives. 1 Sep 1999:139-152

[44] Awasthi S, Nichter M, Pande V. Developing an interactive STD-prevention program for youth: Lessons from a north Indian slum. Studies in Family Planning. 2000;**31**(2):138-150

[45] Klem J, Owens A, Ross A, Edwards L, Cobia DC. Dating violence: Counseling adolescent females from an existential perspective. Journal of Humanistic Counseling, Education and Development. 2009;**48**:48-64

[46] Hays DG, Craigen LM, Knight J, Healey A, Sikes A. Duty to warn and protect against self-destructive behaviors and interpersonal violence. Journal of School Counseling. 2009;**7**(11):11

[47] Carlson LA. Existential theory: Helping school counselors attend to youth at risk for violence. Professional School Counseling. 2003;**6**:310-315

[48] Manjula B, Janardhana N and Nirmala BP, Psycho social profile of adolescent girls in romantic relationship under care and protection of child welfare committee unpublished thesis submitted for the Award of Doctor of Philosophy (Ph. D) in Psychiatric Social Work to the National Institute of Mental Health and Neurosciences (Institute of National Importance), Bengaluru, India